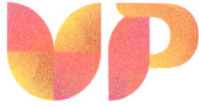

Untold Pilates
Tauranga, New Zealand

Disclaimer

ASPIRATION

In the pages of this book, my aspiration is to ignite a global movement among Pilates instructors and enthusiasts. As you embark on these thoughtfully designed Pilates Reformer routines, my hope is it becomes a catalyst for a new wave of creativity and transformation. Let these progressions not just guide your movements, but also spark your imagination. I believe Pilates is not confined within the reformer's frame; it's a philosophy that empowers us to push boundaries, to invent, and to evolve. Let's enrich it with our unique insights, turning each routine into a canvas for innovation. Together, let us dissolve the boundaries of convention using this book as a stepping stone towards a more collaborative, vibrant, inventive Pilates practice. Allow this book to unite instructors and clients around the globe in a shared journey of movement, growth and inspiration. I hope to inspire and empower instructors around the world, fostering a sense of unity and collective growth within the Pilates community.

FOREWORD

"Arnel's guide is a groundbreaking exploration of Pilates ~ an odyssey beyond the classical confines, into a realm of modifications and variations that will redefine your teaching. In your hands, you hold a passport to unparalleled diversity and innovation within the world of Pilates where you can breathe new life into your everyday practice… Enjoy!"

Tahlia Charleson
Director of The Pilates Fix
Tauranga, New Zealand

Arnel is an exceptional and creative Pilates teacher. His ability to design Reformer progressions while keeping the principles of Pilates woven within his work is inspiring.

This book is a must for any Pilates Group Reformer teachers to help their dedicated long-term clients find even more joy in movement through Pilates. Arnel's passion for the Pilates Method shines through in every page. Reformer instructors will relish this resource. It will help progress your creative spirit and keep the flame of enthusiasm alive in your classes.

Tania Huddart
Owner / Hearts & Bones Pilates
Nelson, New Zealand

I was a client of Arnel for a while, and I truly appreciated his unique teaching approach that embraced creative challenges. This experience played a significant role in motivating me to establish my own studio. So, when I came across the content of this book, it resonated with me completely. It serves as an excellent resource to equip my class with innovation and individuality. I highly recommend it to educators and clients alike who are eager to explore this direction.

Zelda Ruiz
Owner / Pilates Instructor
Pilates Fit & More studio
Cebu, Philippines

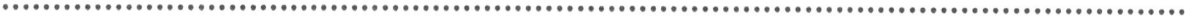

ACKNOWLEDGEMENTS

I am immensely grateful to the individuals who have played an instrumental role in shaping my journey as a Pilates instructor and making this book a reality.

First and foremost, my sincere appreciation goes to my dear friend of three decades, Michel Velasco from Pilates Plus. His early recognition of my potential and patient guidance during the formative years of my career have been invaluable. Without his unwavering support and mentorship, I wouldn't have reached the heights I stand at today.

I extend my deepest gratitude to Ingrid Ramos for her unyielding trust and all-encompassing support. From facilitating my Pilates training to fostering my growth through workshops and seminars, Ingrid's dedication has been a driving force. The creation of Spinework Pilates studio to nurture my aspirations stands as a testament to her belief in me.

I would like to express my gratitude to this lovely couple Barclay and Monika Wilkinson who heartedly supported behind the scenes.

A special mention goes to Tahlia Charleson and the Pilates Fix studio, where I currently serve as a resident senior Pilates instructor. The inspiration and wholehearted support from Tahlia and the studio have been essential, and the captivating images within this book owe their presence to their collaboration.

Lastly, sincere thank you to Tania Huddart from Heart and Bones Pilates studio for disseminating her extensive Pilates knowledge and editing skills. Her expertise has elevated the communication standards on every page of this book. Tania's wealth of experience in book publishing and being a Pilates master trainer combined to form the core of what makes every word and the journey of creating this book invaluable."

C O N T E N T S

UNTOLD PART II

UNTOLD PART III

UNTOLD PART IV

UNTOLD PART V

UNTOLD PART VI

INTRODUCTION

Introducing "The Untold Pilates Progression" – a groundbreaking journey into the world of the Pilates Reformer. Departing from the conventional, this book redefines the approach to Pilates, unveiling a contemporary and innovative perspective that promises to captivate both intermediate and advanced Pilates instructors and enthusiasts alike.

Dedicated to those who seek to infuse their Pilates practice with creativity and excitement, "The Untold Pilates Progression" unveils a treasure trove of uniquely designed routines. These routines are crafted exclusively to the Reformer machine, bringing a fresh dimension to group classes. While the Classical Pilates Method lays the foundation, this book pushes boundaries, encouraging instructors and clients to explore new realms of movement, challenge and enjoyment.

This book is an essential companion for instructors and clients who yearn for more than just a workout – it is a bridge between tradition and innovation. In a world where individual classical training is the norm, "The Untold Pilates Reformer Progression" unlocks the potential of the Reformer machine in a collective setting. It paves the way for trained teachers to broaden their horizons, infusing their teaching practice with dynamic creativity that breathes life into every session.

Join us in this transformative journey as we unlock the untold possibilities of Pilates Reformer progressions. Welcome to a realm where tradition meets innovation, and where group classes are elevated to exhilarating heights through creative expression.

UNTOLD
PART I

THE CROUCHING TIGER I

Strength: Abs

Level: Intermediate   **Repetition:** 8-10   **Springs:** Heavy

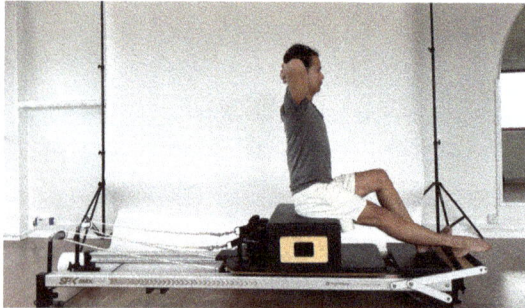

A
START

1. Spine neutral, sitting upright and hands behind the head.
2. One foot hooked under the safety strap, and the other leg extended, on top of the strap.

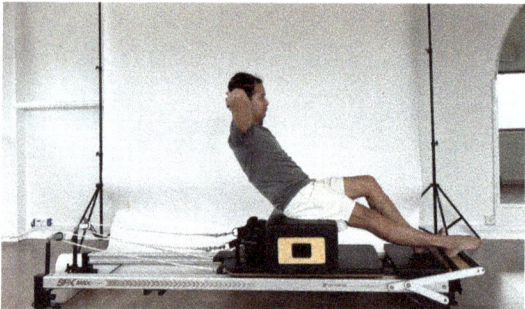

B
EXHALE

1. Roll back half-way.

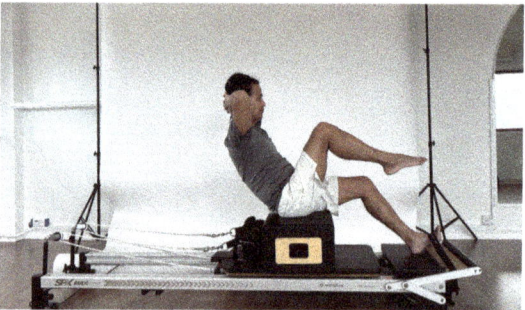

C
INHALE

1. Pull one knee toward your chest .

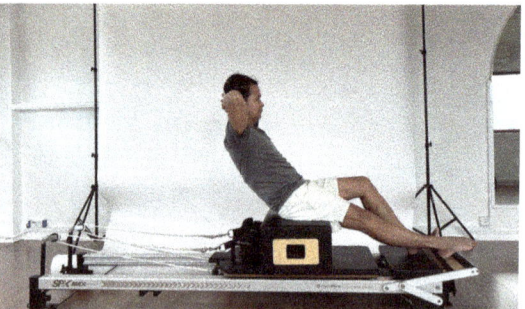

D
EXHALE

1. Return to position **B**.

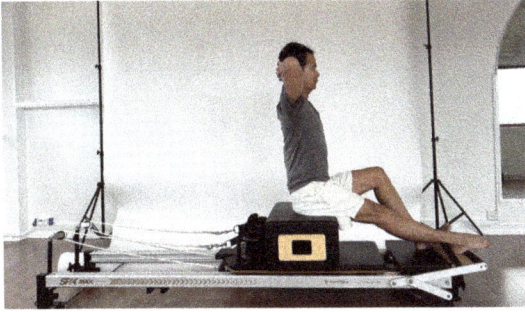

E
INHALE

1. Return to position **A**.
2. Repeat on the other side.

PROGRESSION

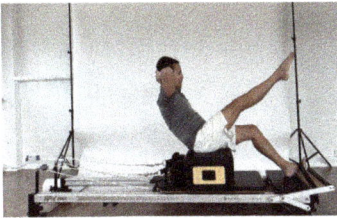

1. Add a straight leg lift **(B)**

THE CROUCHING TIGER II

Strength: Obliques

Level: Intermediate   **Repetition:** 8-10   **Springs:** Heavy

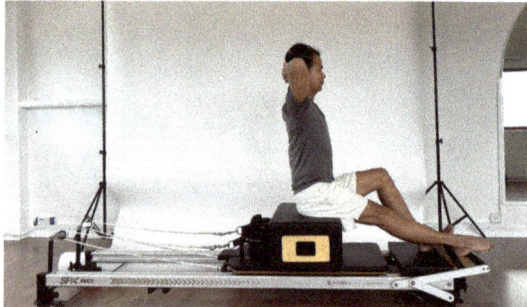

A
START

1. Spine neutral, sitting upright and hands behind your head.
2. One foot hooked under the strap, and other leg extended on top of the strap.

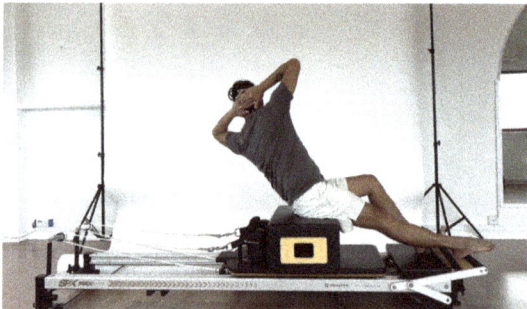

B
EXHALE

1. Twist and lean to the bent leg side.

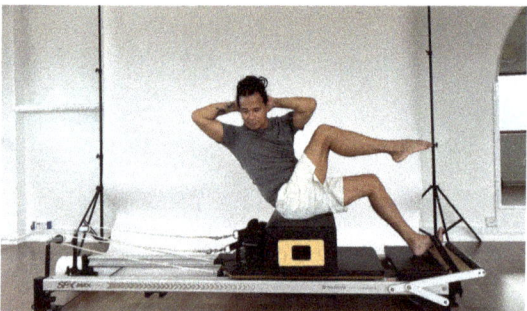

C
EXHALE

1. Twist to the other side while lifting your knee and touching your elbow to the knee.

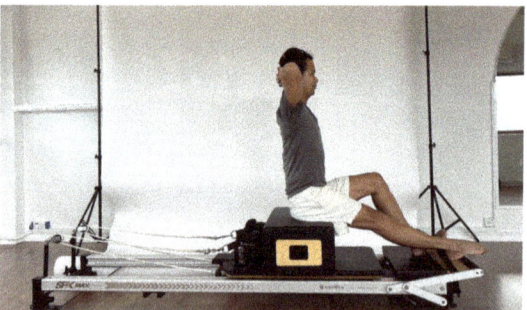

D
INHALE

1. Return to position **A**.
2. Repeat on the other side.

THE CROUCHING TIGER III

Strength: Shoulders, obliques, quads

Level: Intermediate   **Repetition:** 8-10   **Springs:** Heavy

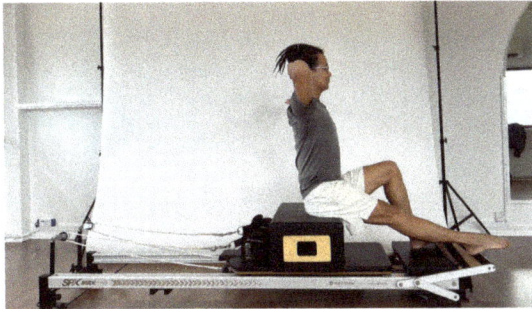

A
START

1. Spine neutral, sitting upright. Place one hand behind your head and the other arm extends out to the side.
2. One foot hooks under the strap, and the other leg is extended and placed on top of the strap.

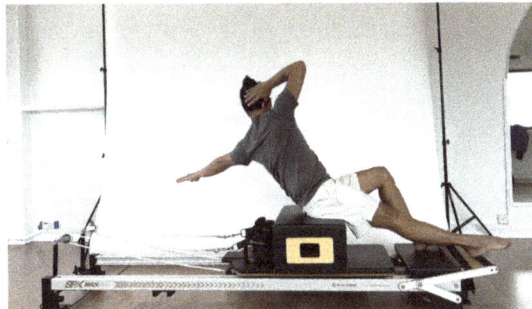

B
INHALE

1. Twist and lean to the bent leg side.

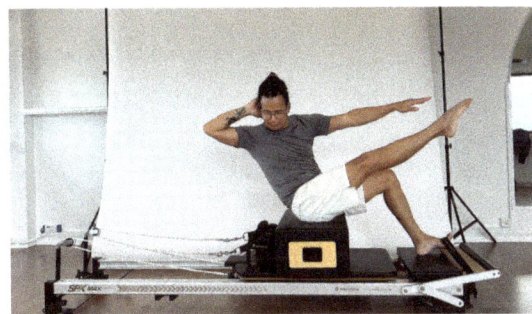

C
EXHALE

1. Lift your straight leg, twist toward the leg and touch your foot with the opposite hand.

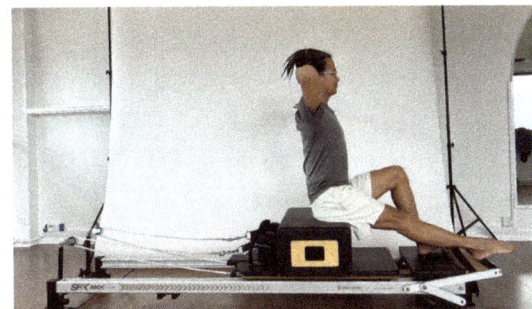

D
INHALE

1. Return to position **A**.
2. Repeat on the other side.

THE FALLING STAR I

Strength: Shoulders, obliques

Level: Intermediate   **Repetition:** 8-10   **Springs:** Heavy

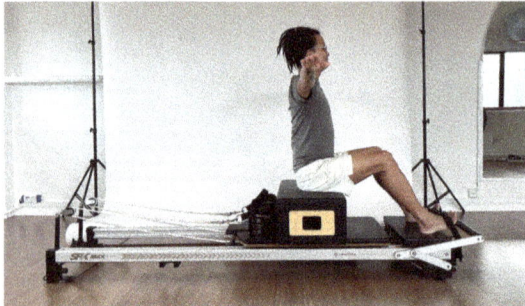

A
START

1. Sit upright with a neutral spine. Stretch both arms out to the side at shoulder level.
2. Place both feet under the strap.

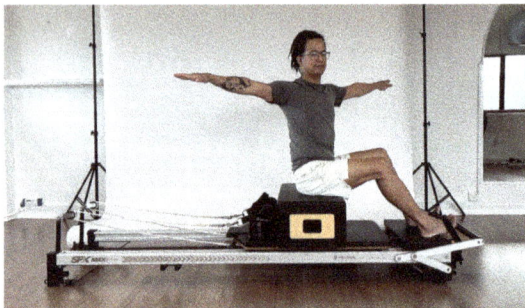

B
INHALE

1. To prepare and exhale as you twist.

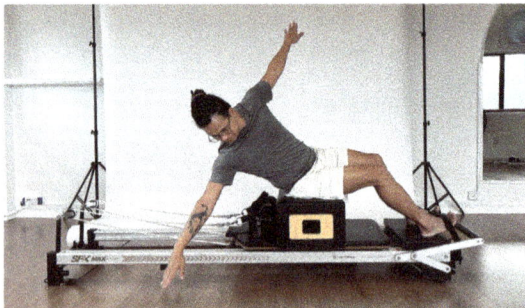

C
EXHALE

1. Lean backward and touch the floor, lift the opposite hip to maintain a neutral spine.

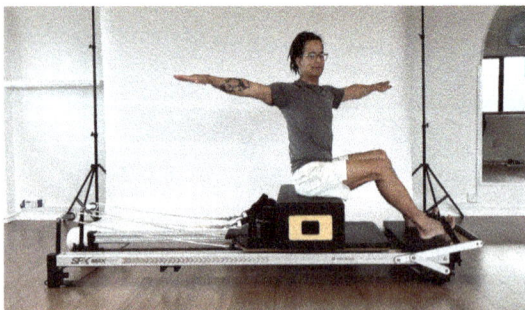

D
INHALE

1. Return to position **B**.

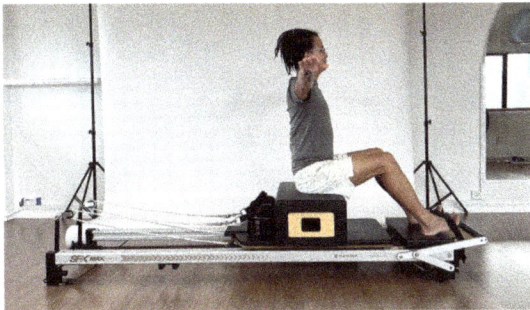

E
EXHALE

1. Return to position **A**.
2. Repeat on the other side.

PROGRESSION 1

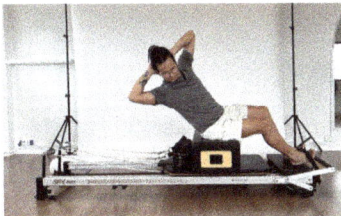

1. Both hands behind head **(C)**

PROGRESSION 2

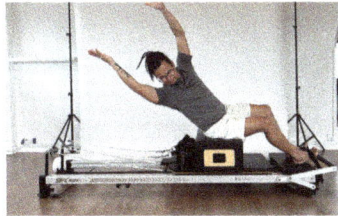

1. Both arms straight over head **(C)**

THE FALLING STAR II

Strength: Shoulders, obliques

Level: Intermediate   **Repetition:** 8-10   **Springs:** Heavy

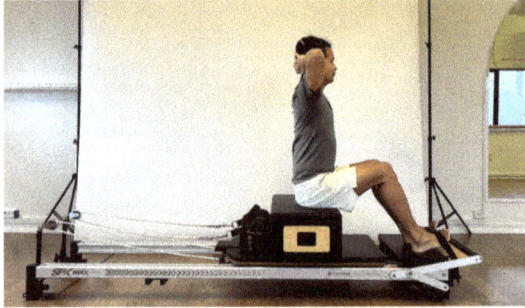

A
START

1. Sit upright in neutral spine with both hands interlaced behind your head.
2. Both feet under the strap.

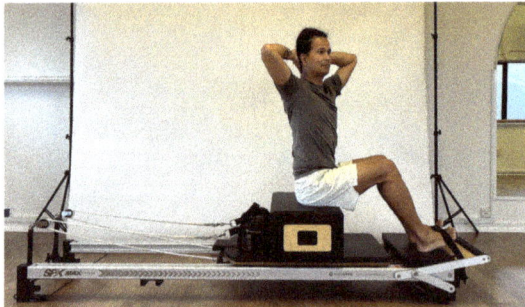

B
INHALE

1. To prepare and exhale as you twist to one side.

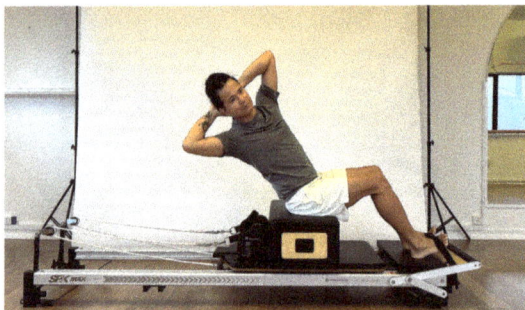

C
EXHALE

1. Lean backward, lifting the opposite hip to maintain a neutral spine.

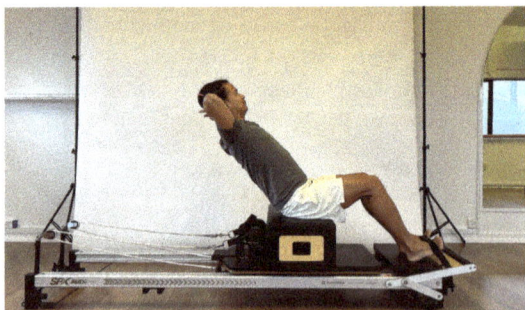

D
INHALE

1. Twist face to ceiling, flexing your spine into a C-curve.

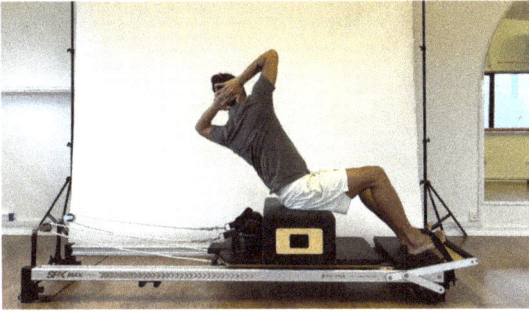

E
EXHALE

1. Rotate to the other side.

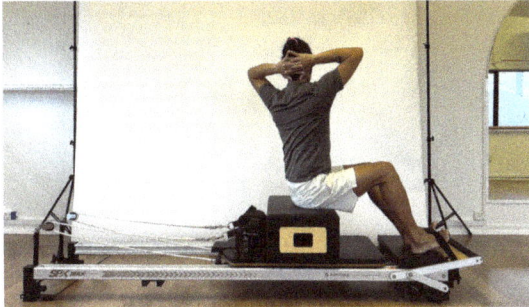

F
INHALE

1. To sit upright maintaining the twist.

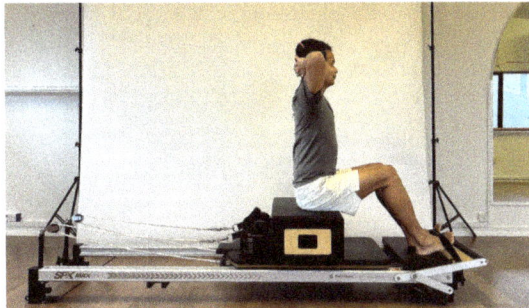

G
EXHALE

1. Return to position **A**.
2. Repeat starting on the other side.

PROGRESSION

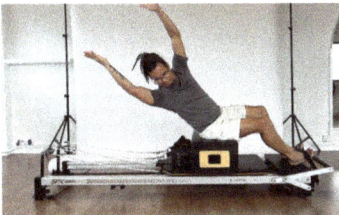

1. Both arms stretch over head **(C)**

AB-BORT I

Strength: Abs, obliques, quads

Level: Advance   **Repetition:** 8-10   **Springs:** Medium

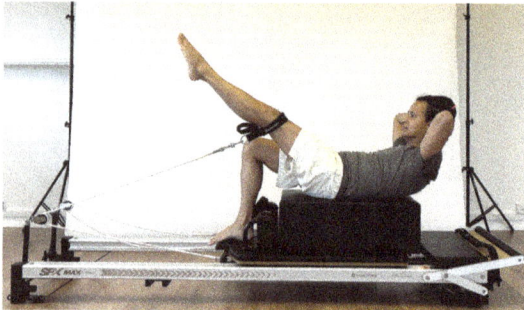

A
START

1. Lie on your back on the box facing the risers in a basic abdominal curl position.
2. Place both hands behind your head supporting your neck.
3. Place one strap above the knee. Extend the leg to 45 degrees. Place the other foot on the headrest.

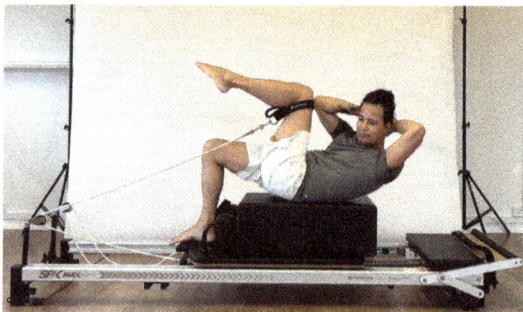

B
EXHALE

1. Twist your trunk and bend your strap leg, bringing the opposite elbow to the knee.

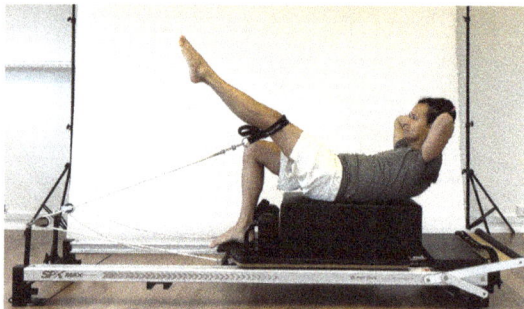

C
INHALE

1. Return to position **A**.
2. Repeat on the other side.

PROGRESSION

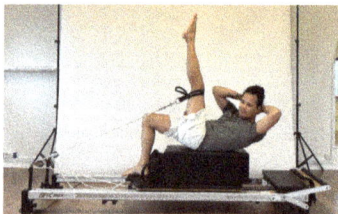

1. Lift your straight leg to 90 degrees as you twist **(B)**

AB-BORT II

Strength: Abs, obliques, quads

Level: Advance   **Repetition:** 8-10   **Springs:** Medium

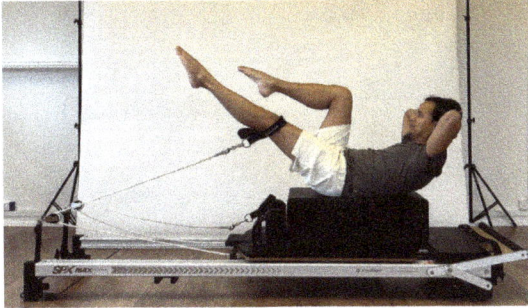

A
START

1. Lie on your back on the box facing the risers in a basic abdominal curl position.
2. Place both hands behind your head supporting your neck.
3. Place one strap above the knee, extending the leg to 45 degrees. Place the other leg in table top.

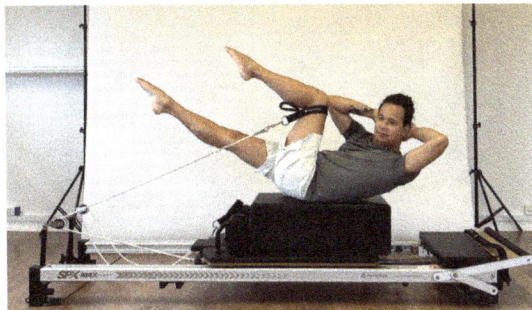

B
EXHALE

1. To bring your strap leg to table top, bring your opposite elbow to the bending knee.
2. Extend the opposite leg out to 45 degrees.

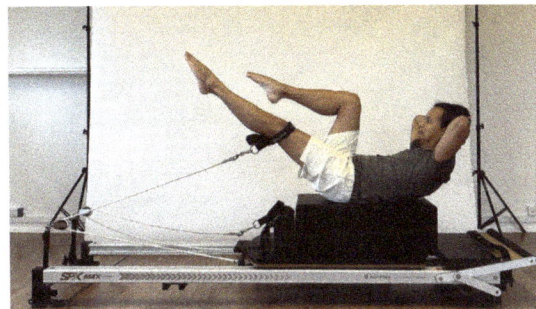

C
INHALE

1. Return to position **A**.
2. Repeat on the other side.

AB-BORT III

Strength: Abs, obliques, quads

Level: Advance   **Repetition:** 8-10   **Springs:** Medium

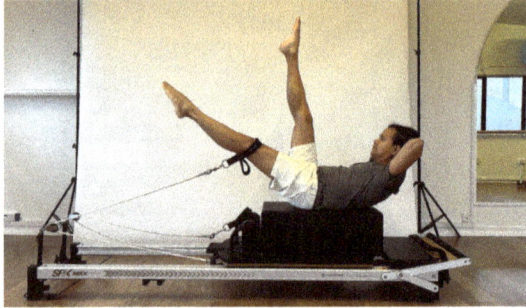

A
START

1. Lie on your back on the box facing the risers in a basic abdominal curl position.
2. Place both hands behind your head supporting your neck.
3. Place one strap above the knee, extending the leg to 45 degrees. Extend the other leg up toward the ceiling at 90 degrees.

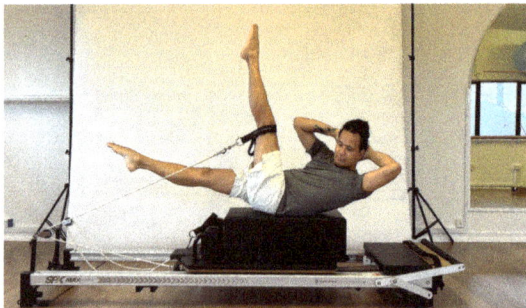

B
EXHALE

1. Lift your strap leg to the ceiling as you twist and bring your opposite elbow to the lifted leg.
2. At the same time lower the elevated leg to 45 degrees.

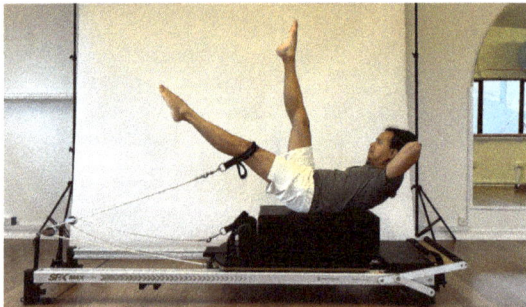

C
INHALE

1. Return to position **A**.
2. Repeat on the other side.

THE NETWORK I

Strength: Biceps, abs, quads, inner thighs

Level: Intermediate   **Repetition:** 8-10   **Springs:** Medium

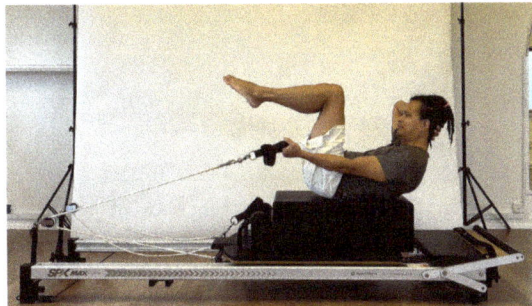

A
START

1. Lie on your back on the box facing the risers in a basic abdominal curl position.
2. Place one hand behind your head. Extend the other arm next to your body and hold the strap.
3. Place both legs in table top.

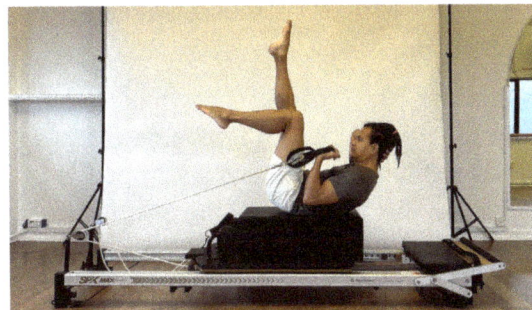

B
EXHALE

1. Bend the elbow of the strap hand, keeping your elbow in the same place.
2. Extend the opposite leg to 90 degrees.

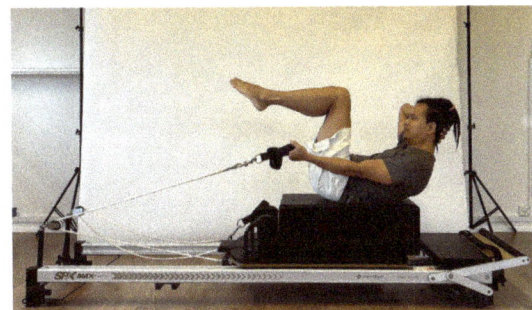

C
INHALE

1. Return to position **A**.
2. Repeat on the other side.

PROGRESSION 1

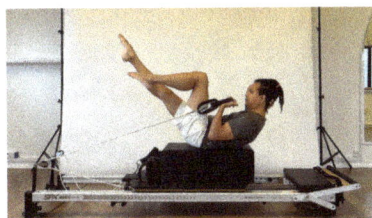

1. Opposite leg extends 45 degrees **(B)**

PROGRESSION 2

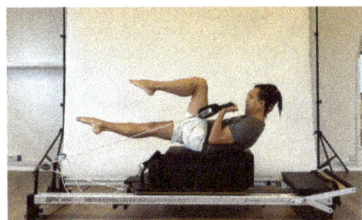

1. Opposite leg extends 180 degrees **(B)**

THE NETWORK II

Strength: Biceps, abs, obliques, quads, inner thighs

Level: Intermediate   **Repetition:** 8-10   **Springs:** Medium

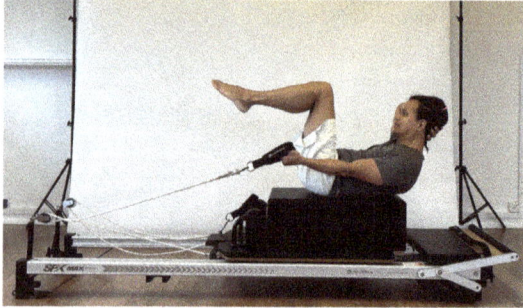

A

START

1. Lie on your back on the box facing the risers in a basic abdominal curl position.
2. Place one hand behind your head. Extend the other arm next to your body and hold the strap.
3. Place both legs in table top.

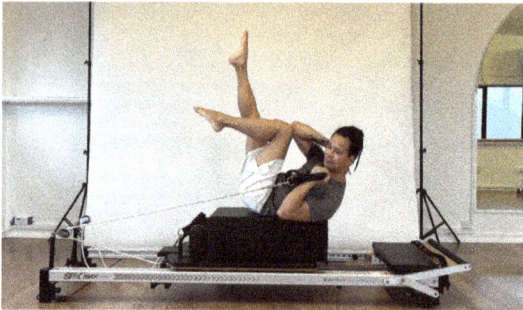

B

EXHALE

1. Bend the elbow of the strap hand, keeping your elbow in the same place.
2. Twist your spine to touch your opposite elbow to the bent leg on the strap side.
3. Extend the opposite leg to 90 degrees.

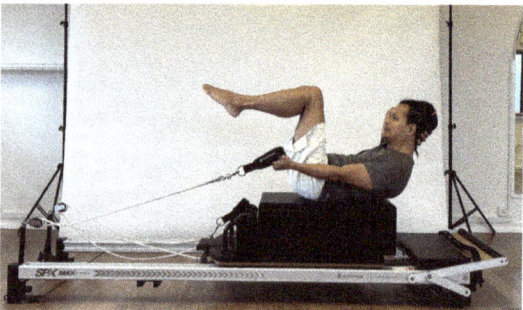

C

INHALE

1. Return to position **A**.
2. Repeat on the other side.

PROGRESSION 1

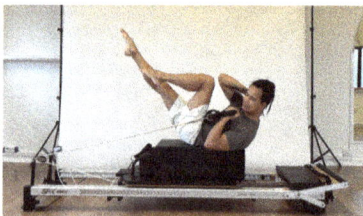

1. Opposite leg extends 45 degrees **(B)**

PROGRESSION 2

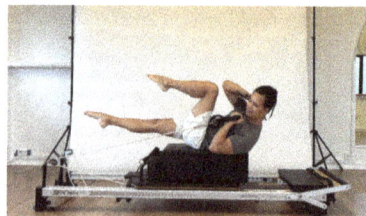

1. Opposite leg extends 180degrees **(B)**

THE EXPANSION

Strength: Biceps, abs, quads, inner thighs,

Level: Intermediate   **Repetition:** 8-10   **Springs:** Medium

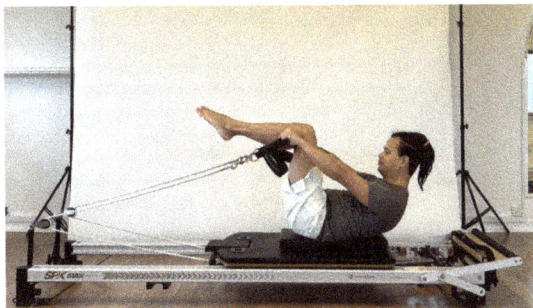

A
START

1. Lie on your back on the box facing the risers in a basic abdominal curl position.
2. Hold the straps in your hands, arms extended to just below shoulder level.
3. Place both legs in table top .

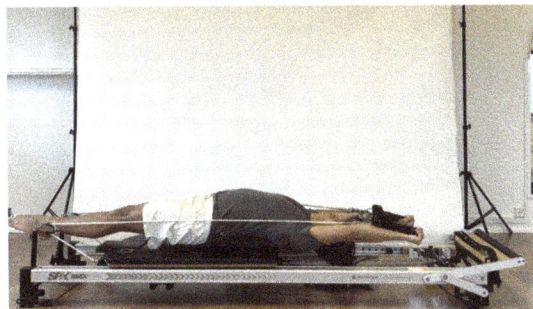

B
EXHALE

1. Extend your legs, arms and spine.
2. Your head lowers behind the box as you bring your arms over your head.

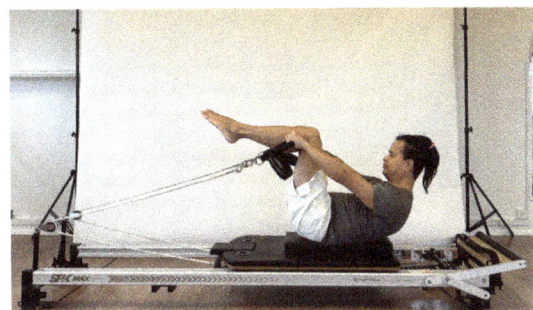

C
INHALE

1. Return to position **A**.

PREFAB I

Strength: arms, lats, abs, quads, inner thighs

Level: Intermediate   **Repetition:** 8-10   **Springs:** Medium

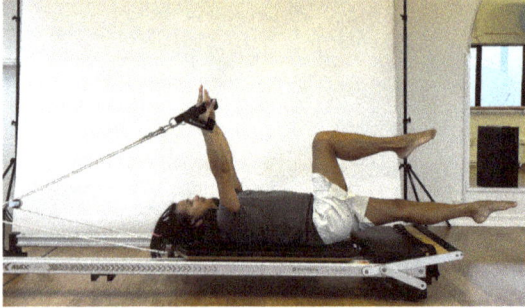

A
START

1. Supine on the carriage.
2. One leg is placed in table top, the other is extended in line with the hip at 180 degrees.
3. Hold the straps in your hands above shoulder level.

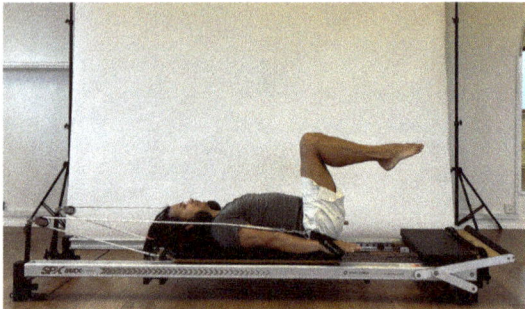

B
EXHALE

1. As you press your hands down to the carriage and bring the extended leg to table top.

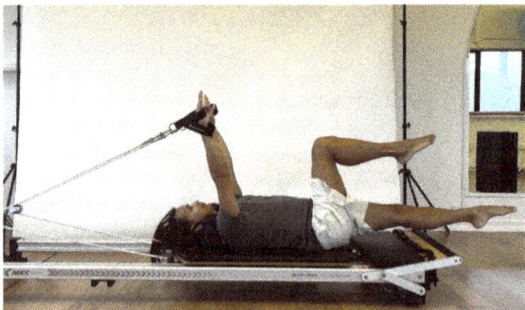

C
INHALE

1. Return to position **A**.
2. Repeat on the other side.

PROGRESSION 1

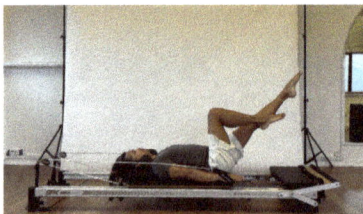

1. Bring the lower leg to 45 degrees **(B)**

PROGRESSION 2

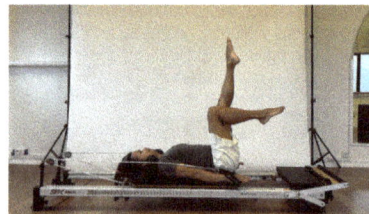

1. Bring the lower leg to 90 degrees **(B)**

PREFAB II

Strength: Arms, lats, abs, quads, inner thighs

Level: Intermediate   **Repetition:** 8-10   **Springs:** Medium

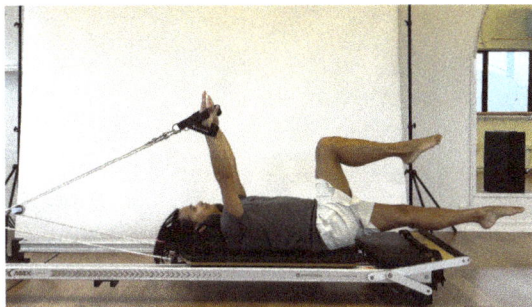

A
START

1. Supine on the carriage.
2. One leg is placed in table top, the other is extended in line with the hip at 180 degrees.
3. Hold the straps in your hands above shoulder level.

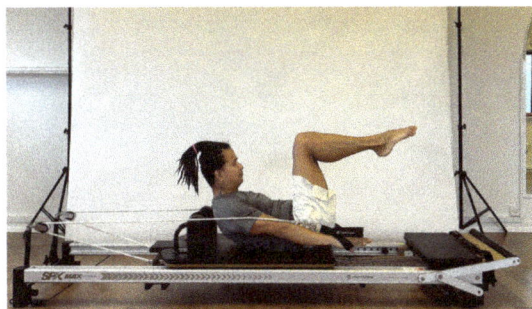

B
EXHALE

1. As you press your hands down to the carriage, lift your head and shoulders up to the abdominal curl position.
2. Bring the extended leg to table top.

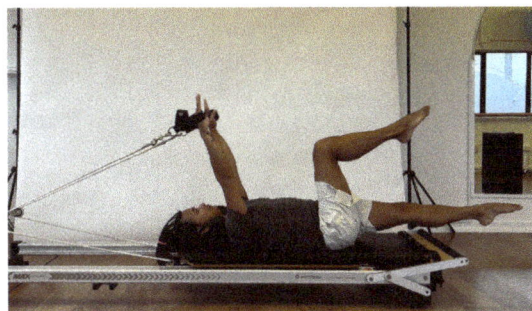

C
INHALE

1. Return to position **A**.

PROGRESSION 1

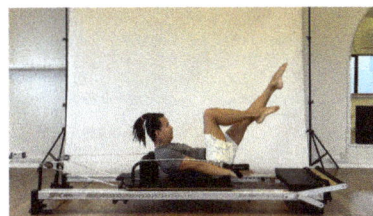

1. Bring the lower leg to 45 degrees **(B)**

PROGRESSION 2

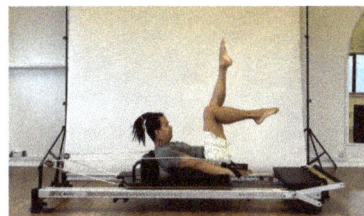

1. Bring the lower leg to 90 degrees **(B)**

PREFAB III

Strength: arms, lats, abs, quads, inner thighs

Level: Intermediate   **Repetition:** 8-10   **Springs:** Medium

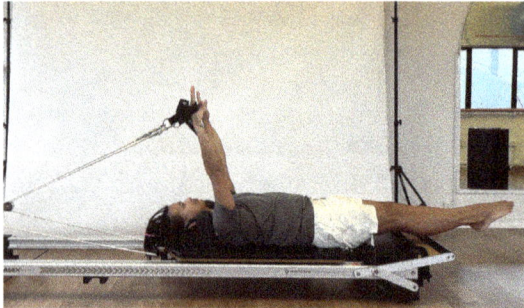

A
START

1. Supine on the carriage.
2. Extend both legs in line with the hips at 180 degrees.
3. Hold the straps in your hands above shoulder level.

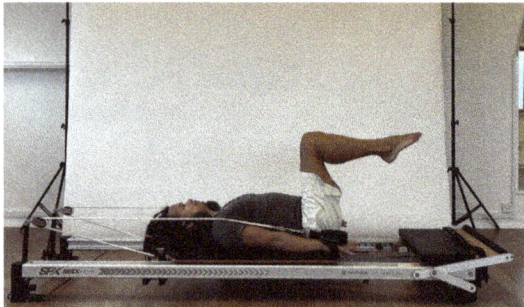

B
EXHALE

1. As you press your hands down to the carriage bring both legs to table top.

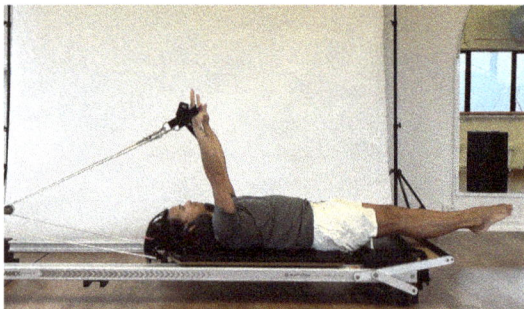

C
INHALE

1. Return to position **A**.

PROGRESSION 1

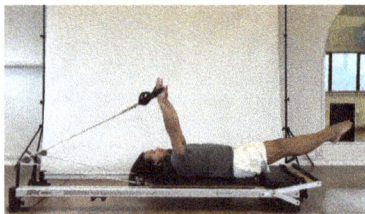

1. Lift both legs just above 180 degrees **(B)**

PROGRESSION 2

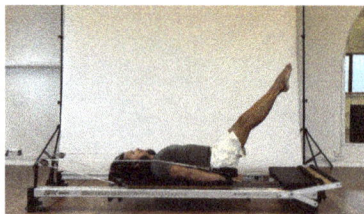

1. Lift both legs to 45 degrees **(B)**

PROGRESSION 3

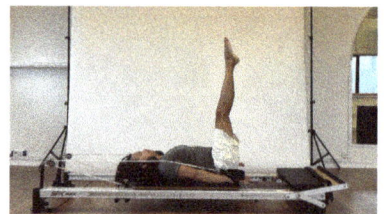

1. Lift both legs to 90 degrees **(B)**

PREFAB IV

Strength: Arms, lats, abs, quads, inner thighs

Level: intermediate   **Repetition:** 8-10   **Springs:** Medium

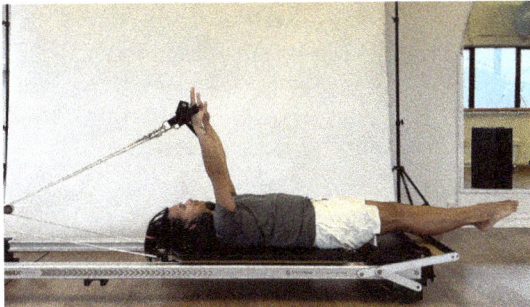

A
START

1. Supine on the carriage.
2. Extend both legs in line with the hips at 180 degrees.
3. Hold the straps in your hands above shoulder level.

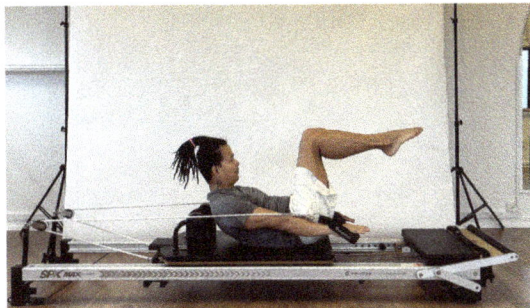

B
EXHALE

1. As you press your hands down to the carriage lift your head and shoulders up.
2. Bring your legs to table top.

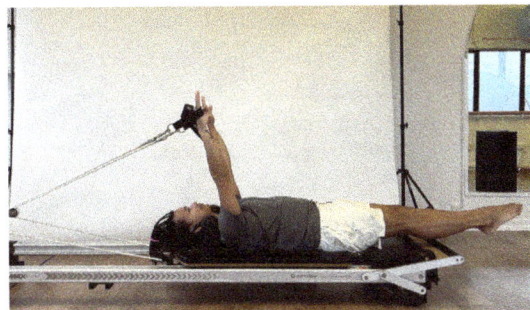

C
INHALE

1. Return to position **A**.

PROGRESSION 1

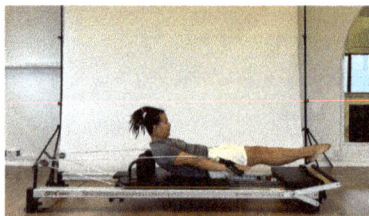

1. Lift both legs to just above 180 degrees **(B)**

PROGRESSION 2

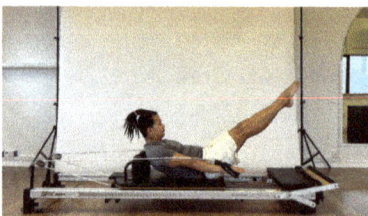

1. Bring both legs to 45 degrees **(B)**

PROGRESSION 3

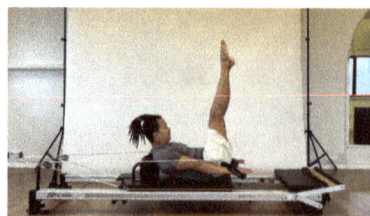

1. Bring both legs to 90 degrees **(B)**

PROGRESSION 4

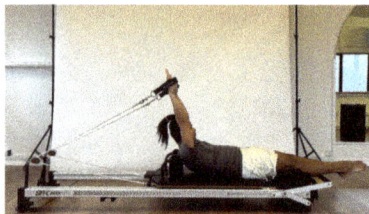

1. Start in the ab curl position and maintain it throughout

THE SPIRAL I

Strength: Chest, shoulders, obliques, quads, inner thighs

Level: Intermediate   **Repetition:** 8-10   **Springs:** Medium

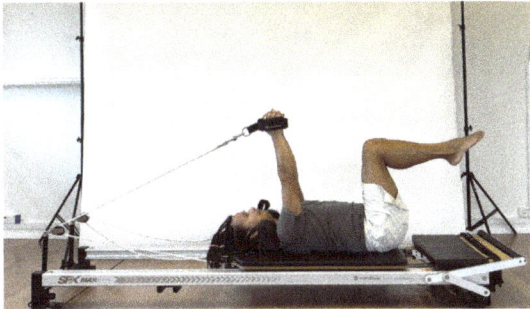

A
START

1. Supine with both legs in table top pressing the legs together.
2. Both hands hold onto one strap.
3. Place the arms just below shoulder level.

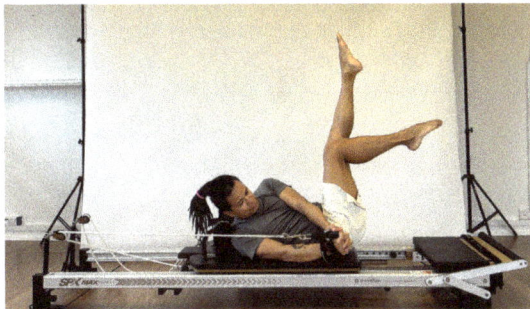

B
EXHALE

1. Pull the strap down toward the hip on the same side as the strap.
2. Your head lifts and rotates together with the chest as you pull the strap.
3. Your opposite leg extends to 90 degrees.

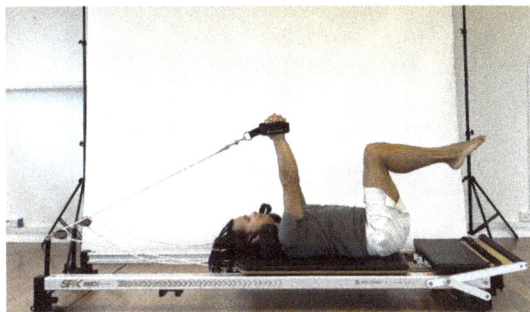

C
INHALE

1. Return to position **A**.
2. Repeat on the other side.

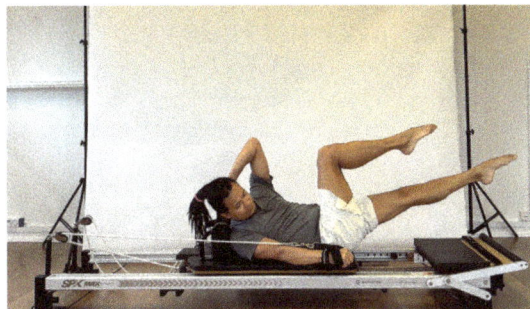

MODIFICATION

1. One hand at the back of the head **B**.

PROGRESSION 1

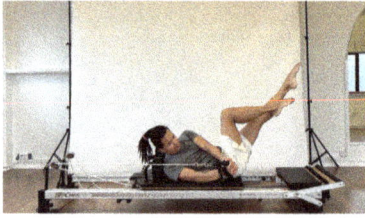

1. Bring the leg to 45 degrees **(B)**

PROGRESSION 2

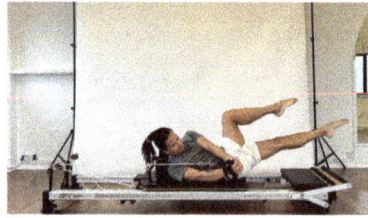

1. Bring the leg to 180 degrees **(B)**

THE SPIRAL II

Strength: Chest, shoulders, obliques, quads, inner thighs

Level: Intermediate   **Repetition:** 8-10   **Springs:** Medium

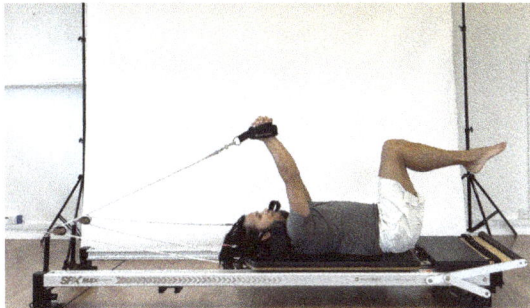

A
START

1. Supine with both legs in table top pressing the legs together.
2. Both hands hold onto one strap.
3. Place the arms just below shoulder level.

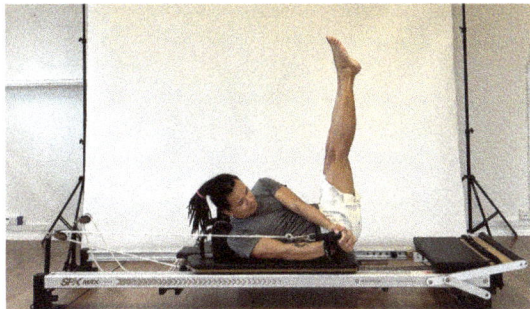

B
EXHALE

1. Pull the strap down toward the hip on the same side as the strap.
2. Your head lifts and rotates together with the chest as you pull the strap.
3. Both legs extend to 90 degrees.

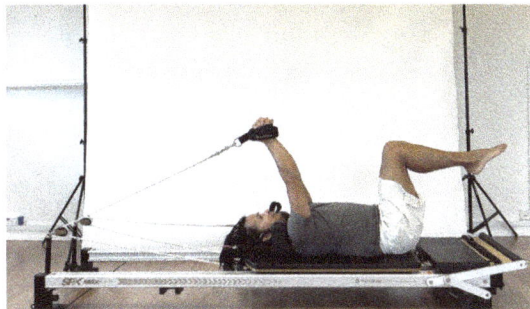

C
INHALE

1. Return to position **A**.
2. Repeat on the other side.

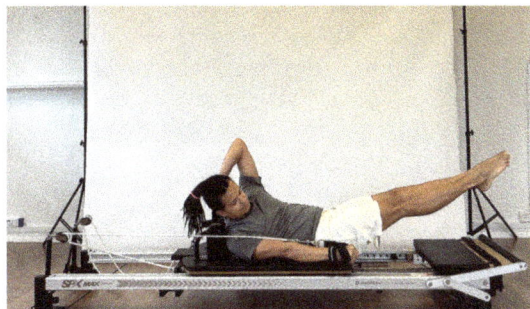

MODIFICATION

1. One hand at the back of the head **B**.

PROGRESSION 1

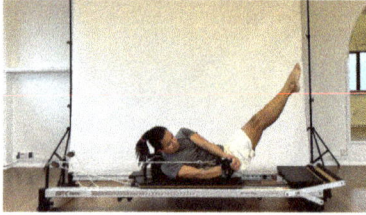

1. Extend both legs to 45 degrees **(B)**

PROGRESSION 2

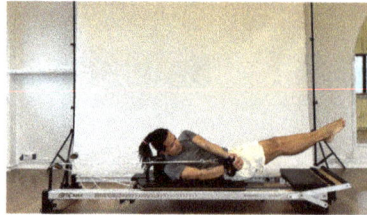

1. Bring the leg to 180 degrees **(B)**

THE SPIRAL III

Strength: Chest, shoulders, oblique, quads, inner thighs

Level: Intermediate   **Repetition:** 8-10   **Springs:** Medium

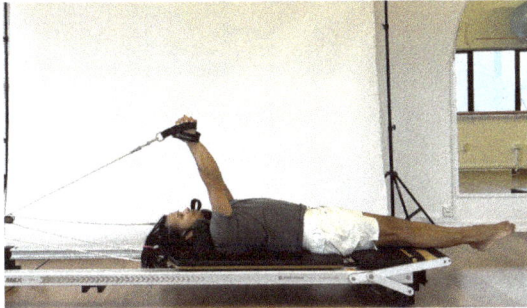

A
START

1. Supine with both legs extended and in line with the hips.
2. Both hands hold onto one strap.
3. Place the arms just below shoulder level.

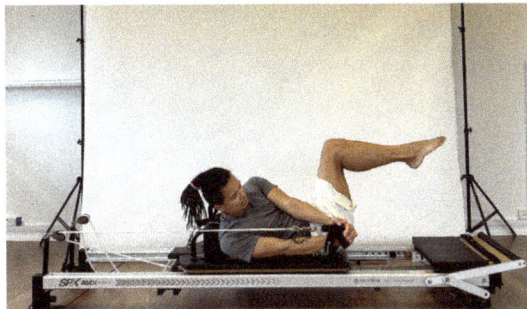

B
EXHALE

1. Pull the strap down toward the hip on the same side as the strap.
2. Your head lifts and rotates together with the chest as you pull the strap.
3. Both legs bend up to table top.

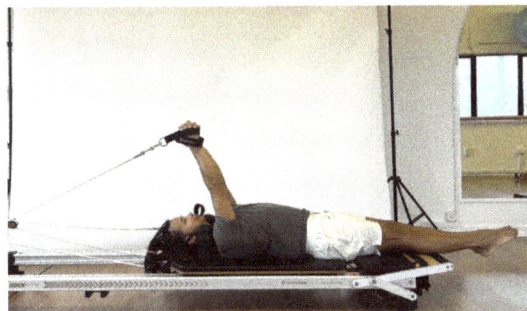

C
INHALE

1. Return to position **A**.
2. Repeat on the other side.

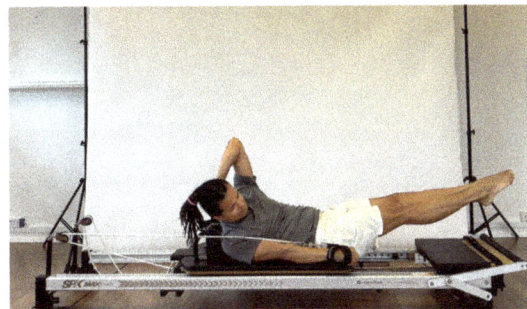

MODIFICATION

1. One hand at the back of the head **B**.

PROGRESSION 1

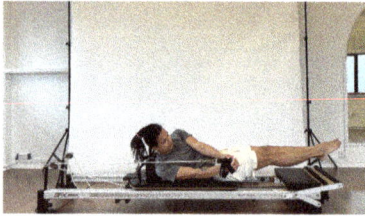

1. Lift the legs to just above 180 degrees **(B)**

PROGRESSION 2

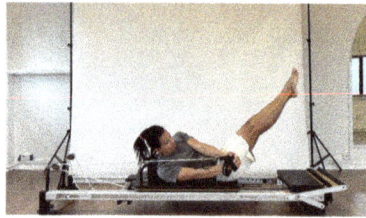

1. Lift the legs to 45 degrees **(B)**

PROGRESSION 3

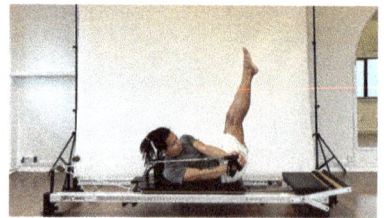

1. Lift the legs to 90 degrees **(B)**

UNTOLD
PART II

CAT STRETCH I

Strength: Chest, shoulders, abs, quads

Level: Intermediate   **Repetition:** 8-10   **Springs:** Medium to light

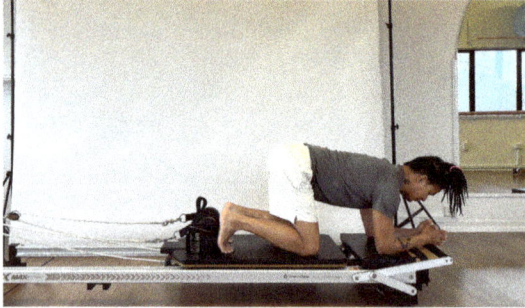

A
START

1. Four point kneel with your feet pressed against the shoulder rests and forearms on the standing platform.
2. Spine in neutral.

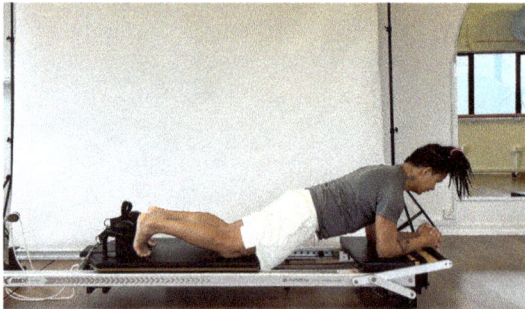

B
EXHALE

1. Extend your legs out behind you keeping your shoulders where they are.
2. Your pelvis tucks under slightly to protect your lower back.

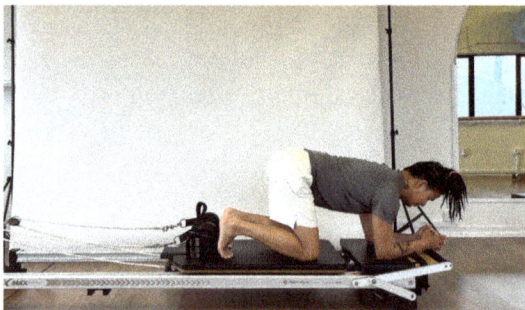

C
INHALE

1. Return to position **A**.

PROGRESSION 1

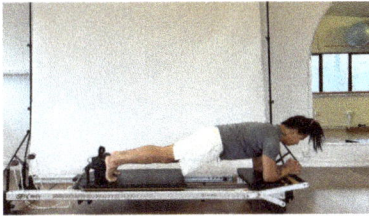

1. Knees off **(B)**

PROGRESSION 2

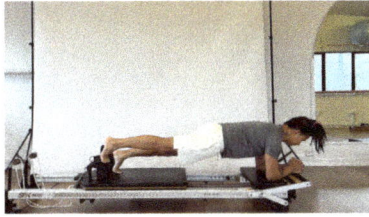

1. One foot on top of the shoulder rest **(B)**

PROGRESSION 3

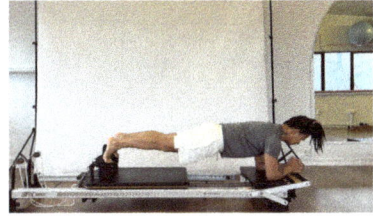

1. Both feet on top of the shoulder rests **(B)**

PROGRESSION 4

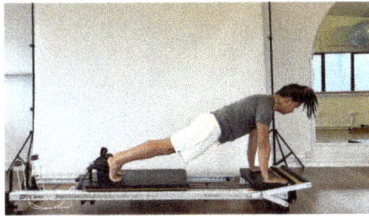

1. Plank position on your hands **(B)**

PROGRESSION 5

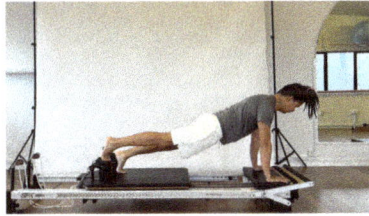

1. One foot on top of the shoulder rest **(B)**

PROGRESSION 6

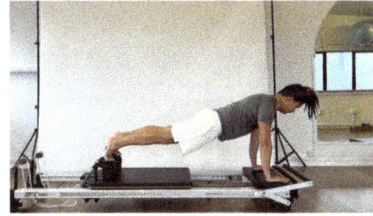

1. Both feet on top of the shoulder rests **(B)**

PROGRESSION 7

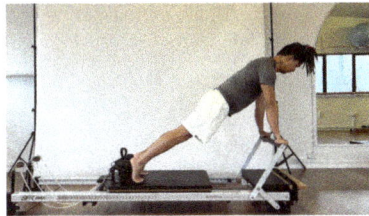

1. Plank position with your hands on the footbar **(B)**

PROGRESSION 8

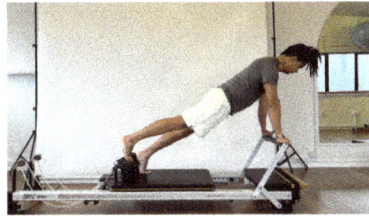

1. One foot on top of the shoulder rest **(B)**

PROGRESSION 9

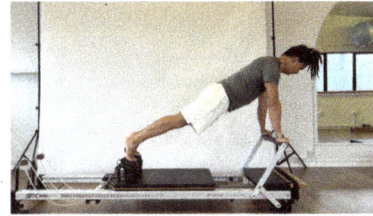

1. Both feet on top of the shoulder rests **(B)**

MODIFICATION

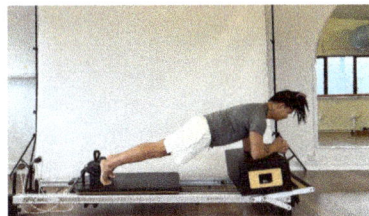

1. Forearms on top of the box **(B)**

CAT STRETCH II

Strength: Chest, shoulder, abs, quads

Level: Intermediate   **Repetition:** 8-10   **Springs:** Medium to light

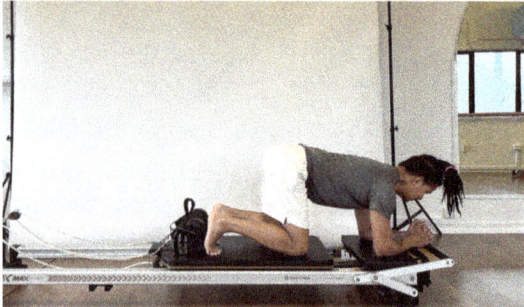

A
START

1. Four point kneel with your feet pressed against the shoulder rests and forearms on the standing platform.
2. Spine in neutral.

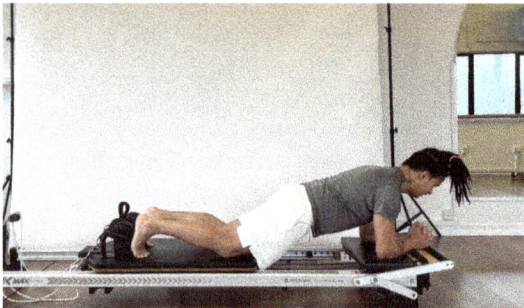

B
EXHALE

1. Extend your legs out behind you. Your knees stay in contact with the carriage.

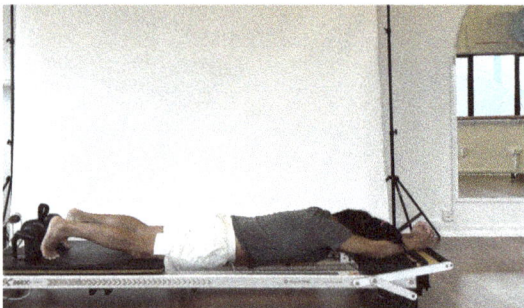

C
INHALE

1. Push the carriage out further, lengthening your arms. Keep your forearms in contact with the standing platform.

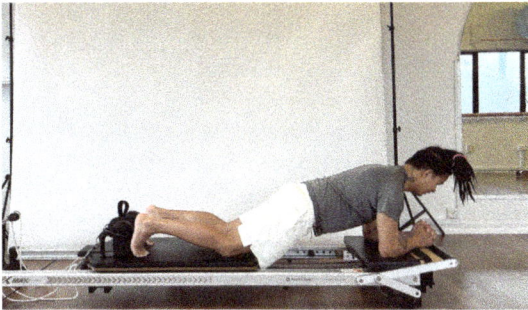

D

EXHALE

1. Return to position **B**.

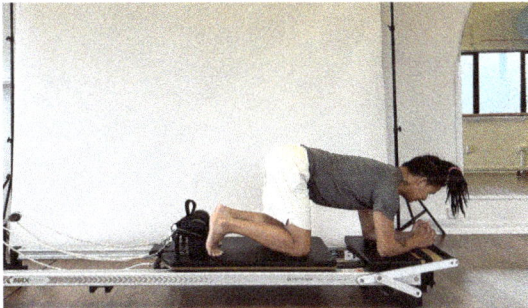

E

INHALE

1. Return to position **A**.

PROGRESSION 1

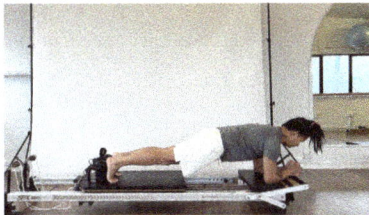

1. Knees off **(B)**

PROGRESSION 2

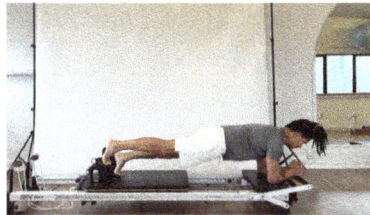

1. One foot on top of the shoulder rest **(B)**

PROGRESSION 3

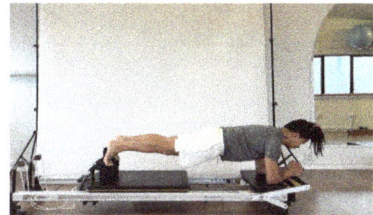

1. Both feet on top of the shoulder rests **(B)**

PROGRESSION 4

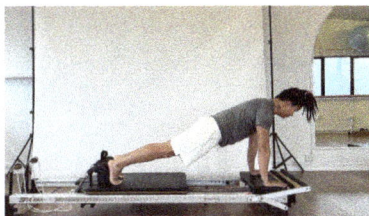

1. Plank position on your hands. Knees off **(B)**

PROGRESSION 5

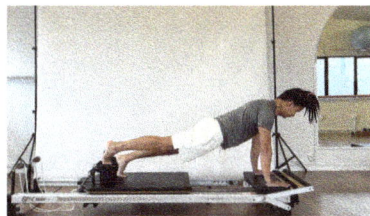

1. One foot on top of the shoulder rest **(B)**

PROGRESSION 6

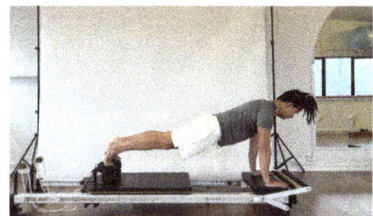

1. Both feet on top of the shoulder rests **(B)**

PROGRESSION 7

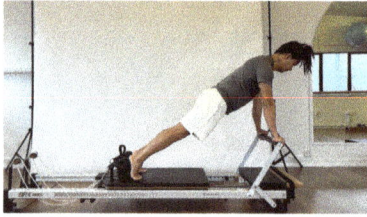

1. Hands on footbar **(B)**

PROGRESSION 8

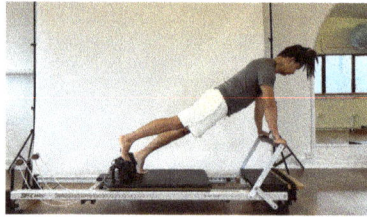

1. One foot on top of the shoulder rest **(B)**

PROGRESSION 9

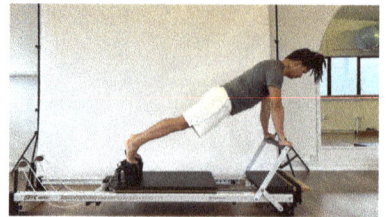

1. Both feet on top of the shoulder rests **(B)**

MODIFICATION

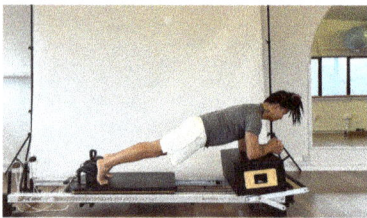

1. Forearms on top of the box **(B)**

CAT STRETCH III

Strength: Chest, shoulders, abs, quads

Level: Intermediate   **Repetition:** 8-10   **Springs:** Medium to light

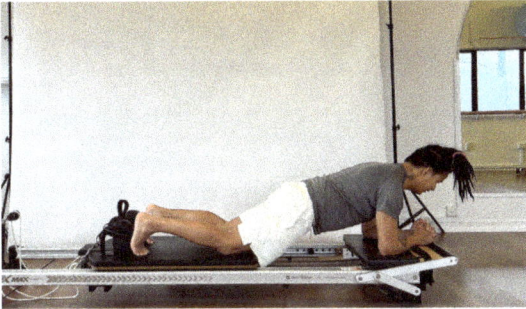

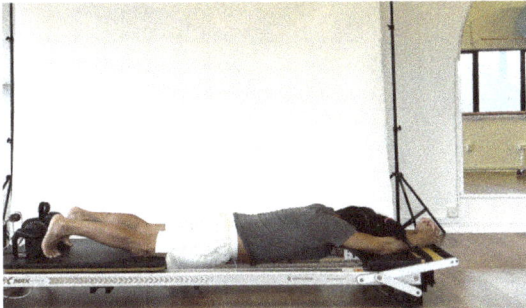

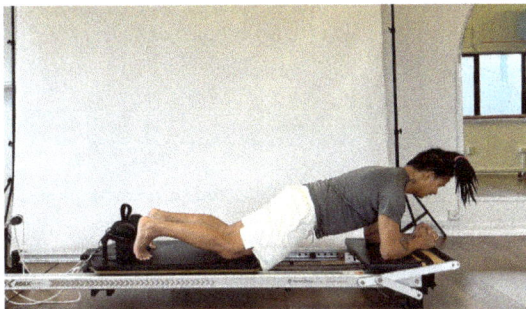

A
START

1. Kneeling plank position, with your forearms on the standing platform.
2. Feet are pressed against the shoulder rests.

B
EXHALE

1. Extend your arms pushing the carriage further back.

C
INHALE

1. Return to position **A**.

PROGRESSION 1

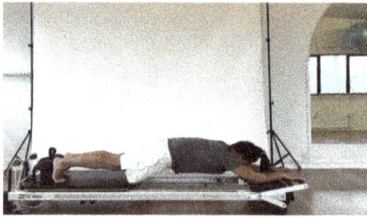

1. Both knees off **(B)**

PROGRESSION 2

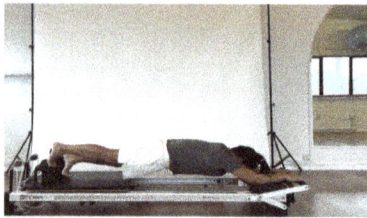

1. One foot on top of the shoulder rest **(B)**

PROGRESSION 3

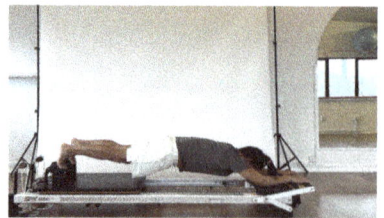

1. Both feet on top of the shoulder rest **(B)**

PROGRESSION 4

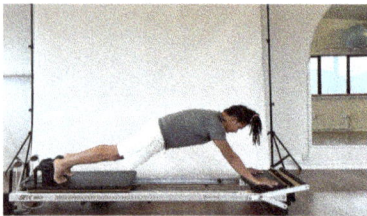

1. Full plank position with your knees off **(B)**

PROGRESSION 5

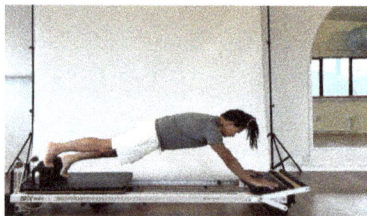

1. One foot on top of the shoulder rest **(B)**

PROGRESSION 6

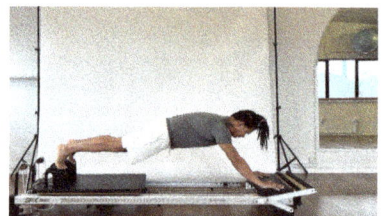

1. Both feet on top of the shoulder rests **(B)**

PROGRESSION 7

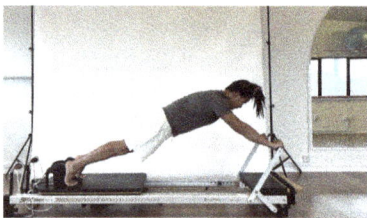

1. Full plank with your hands on the footbar **(B)**

PROGRESSION 8

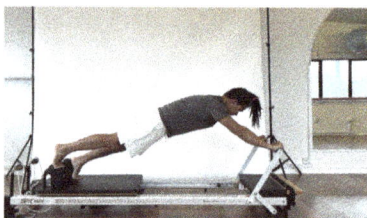

1. One foot on top of the shoulder rest **(B)**

PROGRESSION 9

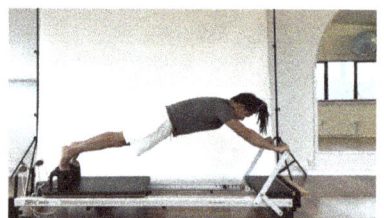

1. Both feet on top of the shoulder rests **(B)**

MODIFICATION

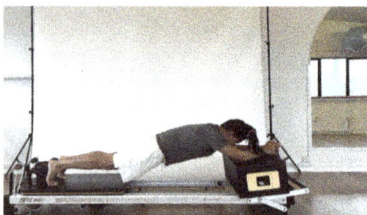

1. Forearms on the box **(B)**

FLYING SQUIRREL I

Strength: Chest, shoulders, abs, quads, glutes

Level: Intermediate   **Repetition:** 8-10   **Springs:** Medium to light

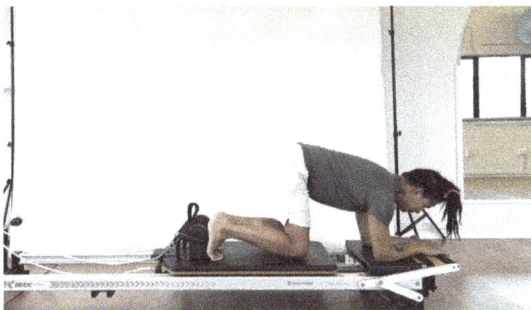

A
START

1. Four point kneel with your feet pressed against the shoulder rests and forearms on the standing platform.
2. Knees are off the carriage.
3. Spine in neutral.

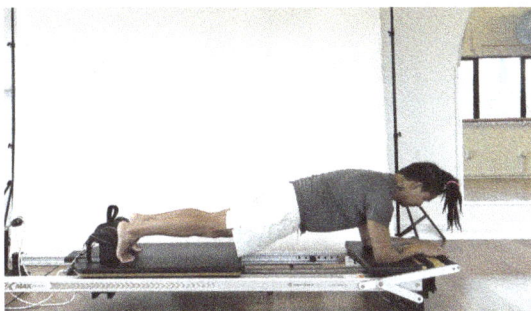

B
EXHALE

1. Extend your legs out, keeping your knees off.

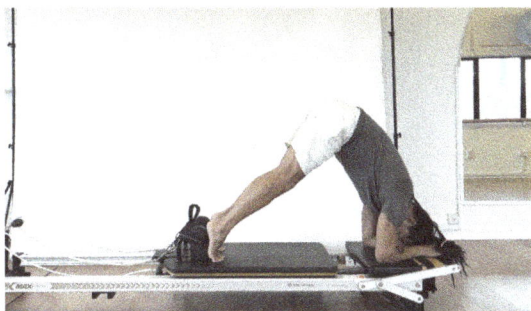

C
INHALE

1. To bring hips up to the ceiling.

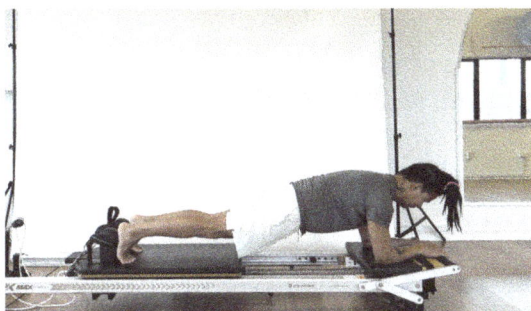

D
EXHALE

1. Return to position **B**.

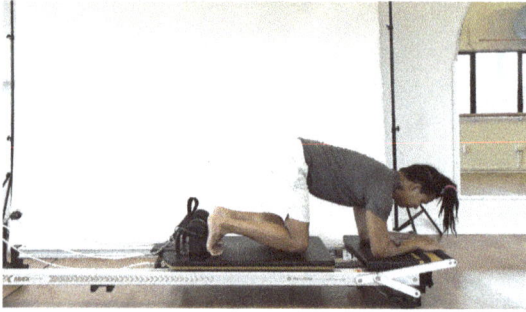

E

INHALE

1. Return to position **A**.

PROGRESSION 1

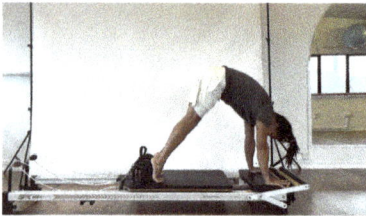

1. Full plank position **(C)**

PROGRESSION 2

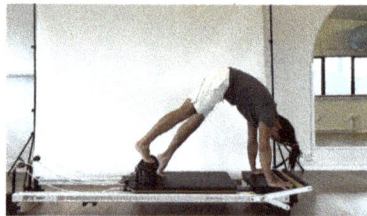

1. One foot on top of the shoulder rest **(C)**

PROGRESSION 3

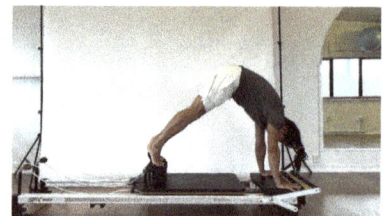

1. Both feet on top of the shoulder rests **(C)**

PROGRESSION 4

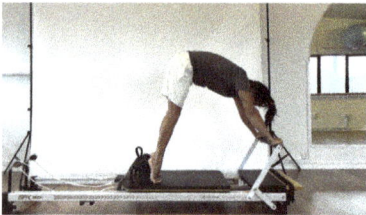

1. Hands on footbar **(C)**

PROGRESSION 5

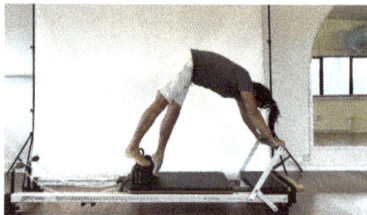

1. One foot on top of the shoulder rest **(C)**

PROGRESSION 6

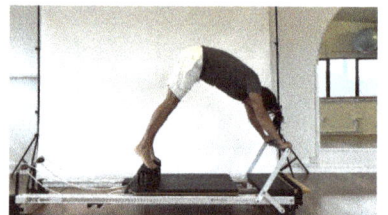

1. Both feet on top of the shoulder rests **(C)**

MODIFICATION

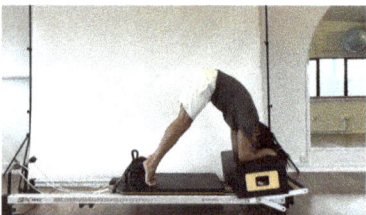

1. Forearms on top of the box **(C)**

FLYING SQUIRREL II

Strength: Chest, shoulders, abs, quads

Level: Intermediate   **Repetition:** 8-10   **Springs:** Medium to light

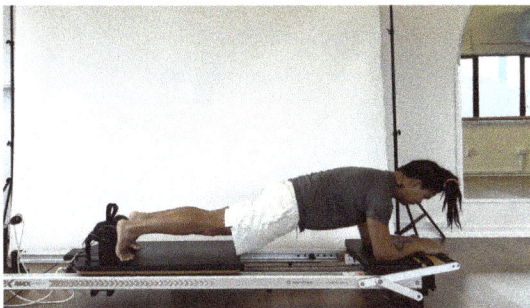

A
START

1. Full plank position, on your forearms.
2. Feet flex against the shoulder rests.

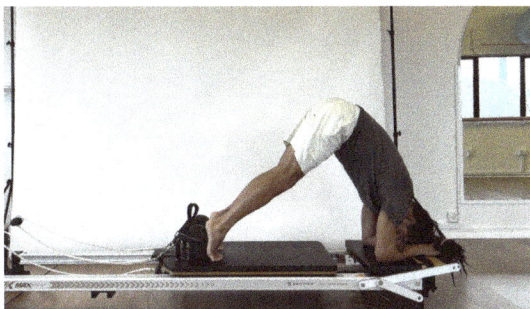

B
EXHALE

1. Lift your hips up to the ceiling.

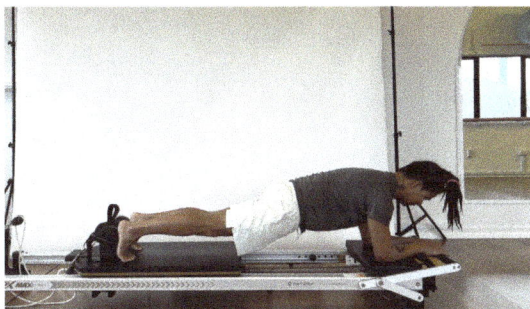

C
INHALE

1. Return to position **A**.

PROGRESSION 1

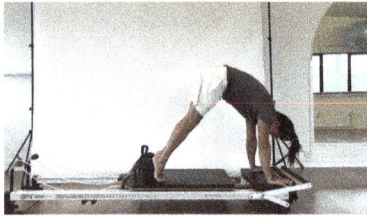

1. Full plank **(B)**

PROGRESSION 2

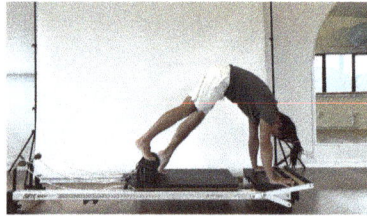

1. One foot on top of the shoulder rest **(B)**

PROGRESSION 3

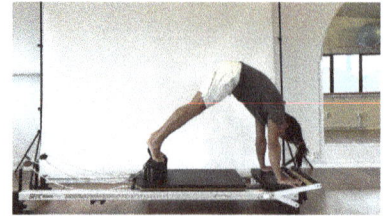

1. Both feet on top of the shoulder rests **(B)**

PROGRESSION 4

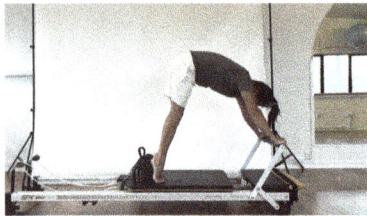

1. Hands on the footbar **(B)**

PROGRESSION 5

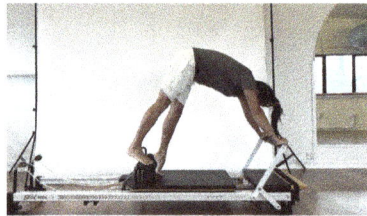

1. One foot on top of the shoulder rest **(B)**

PROGRESSION 6

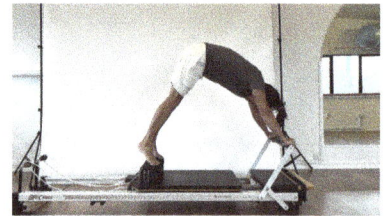

1. Both feet on top of the shoulder rests **(B)**

MODIFICATION

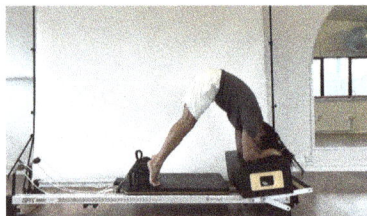

1. Forearms on top of the box **(B)**

FLYING SQUIRREL III

Strength: Chest, shoulders, abs, quads, glutes, hamstrings

Level: Advance   **Repetition:** 8-10   **Springs:** Medium to light

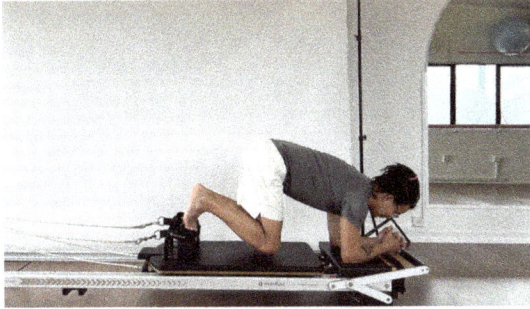

A
START

1. Four point kneel with your feet on top of the shoulder rests and forearms on the standing platform.
2. Knees are off the carriage.
3. Spine in neutral.

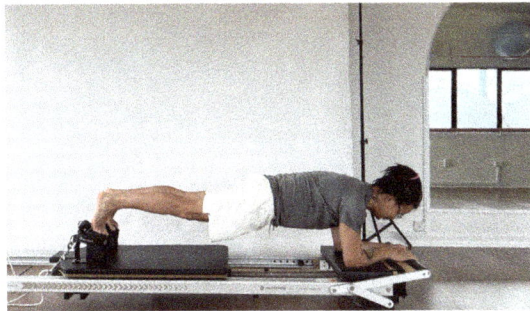

B
EXHALE

1. Extend your legs out keeping your knees off the carriage.

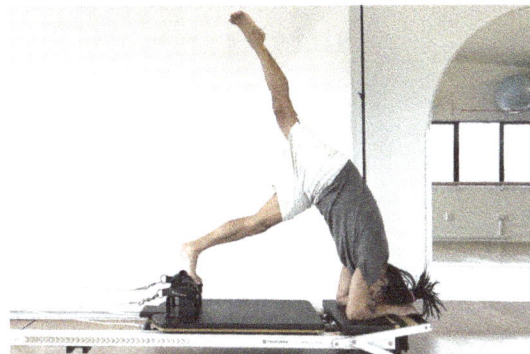

C
INHALE

1. Lift both your hips and one leg (arabesque) up toward the ceiling.

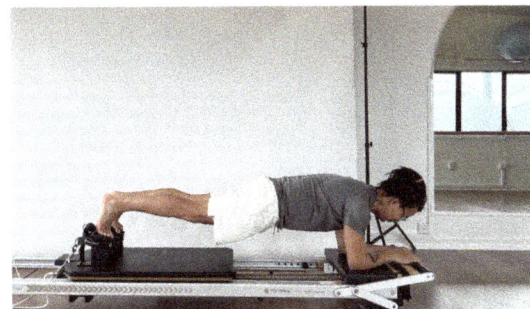

D
EXHALE

1. Return to position **B**.

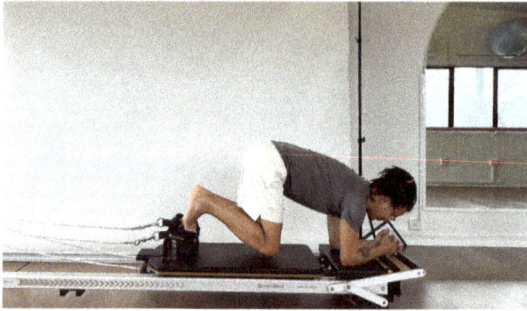

E
INHALE

1. Return to the starting position.
2. Repeat on the other side.

PROGRESSION 1

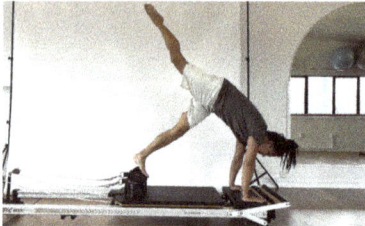

1. Place your hands on the standing platform. Elbows straight **(C)**

PROGRESSION 2

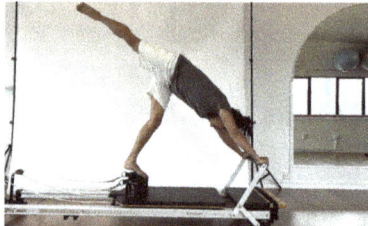

1. Hands on the footbar **(C)**

MODIFICATION

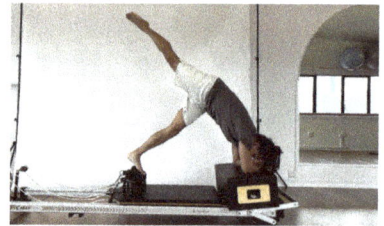

1. Forearms on top of the box **(C)**

FLYING SQUIRREL IV

Strength: Chest, shoulders, abs, quads, glutes, hamstrings

Level: Advance   **Repetition:** 8-10   **Springs:** Medium to light

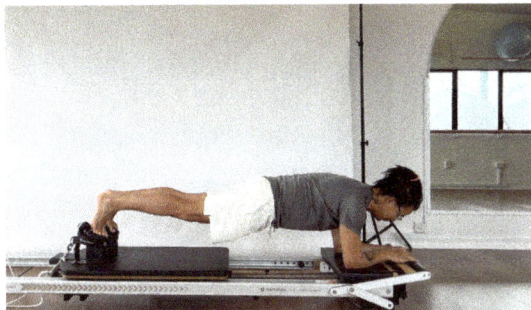

A
START

1. Plank position on your forearms.
2. Place both feet on top of the shoulder rests.
3. Extend both legs out behind you.

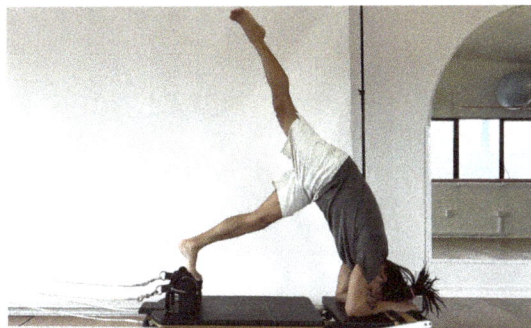

B
EXHALE

1. Lift both your hips and one leg up to the ceiling.

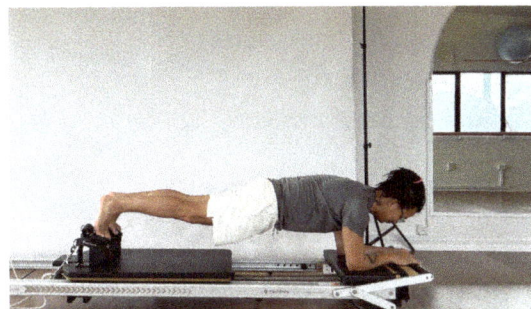

C
INHALE

1. Return to position **A**.
2. Repeat to the other side.

PROGRESSION 1

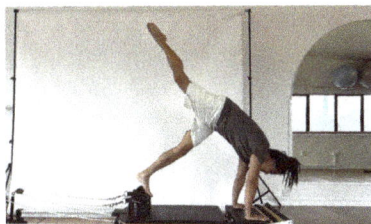

1. Hands on the standing platform with straight arms **(B)**

PROGRESSION 2

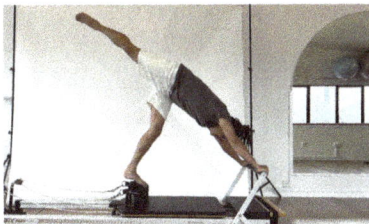

1. Hands on the footbar **(B)**

MODIFICATION

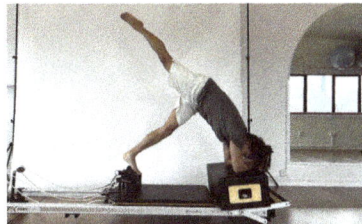

1. Forearms on top of the box **(B)**

THREE TOED SLOTH I

Strength: Chest, shoulders, arms, abs, quads, glutes, hamstrings

Level: Intermediate   **Repetition:** 8-10   **Springs:** Medium to light

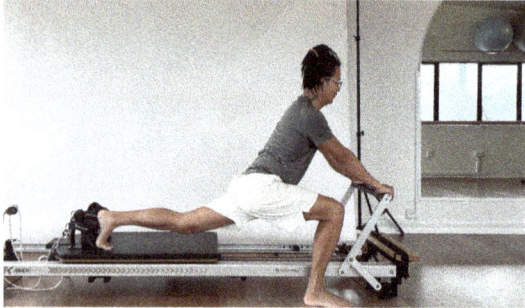

A
START

1. Scooter position, hands on footbar.
2. Outer leg on the floor below shoulder.
3. Inner leg straight, with the foot against the shoulder rest, toes flexed.

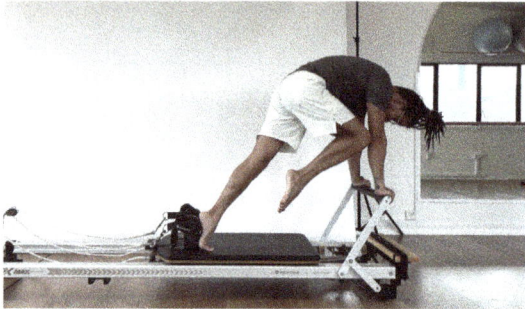

B
EXHALE

1. To pike up - Close the carriage as you lift the foot off the floor, bringing the knee up to the elbow on the same side.
2. Curve your spine.

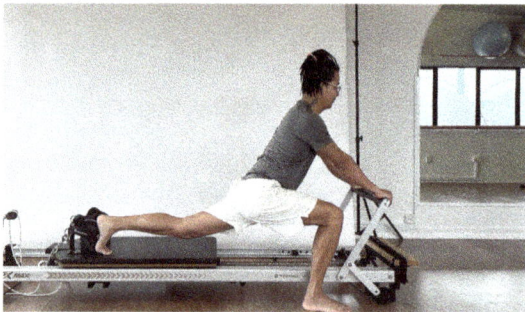

C
INHALE

1. Return position **A**.
2. Repeat on the other side.

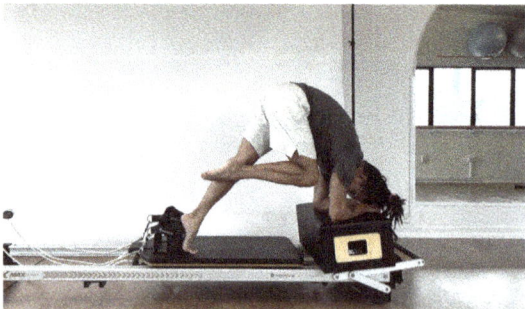

MODIFICATION

1. Forearms on top of the box.

THREE TOED SLOTH II

Strength: Chest, shoulders, arms, abs, quads, glutes, hamstring

Level: Intermediate   **Repetition:** 8-10   **Springs:** Medium to light

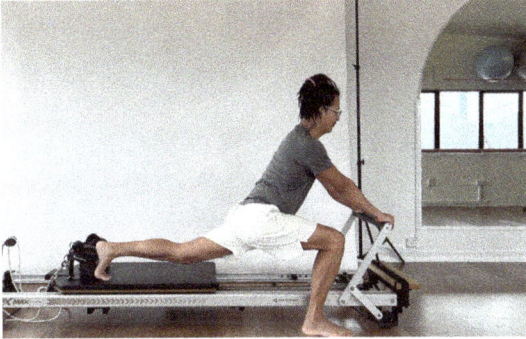

A
START

1. Scooter position, hands on the footbar
2. Place your outer leg on the floor below your shoulder. Bend the knee as you extend the inner leg.
3. The inner leg extends behind you with your toes tucked under against the shoulder rest.

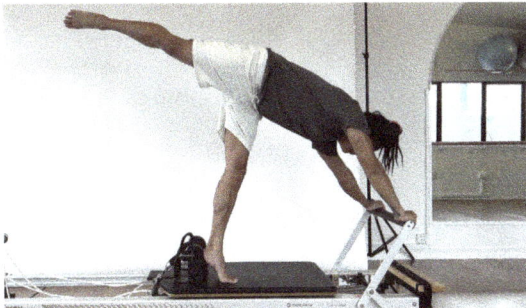

B
EXHALE

1. Push the floor leg up as you lift the leg behind you. Close the carriage at the same time. Your arms support you as your leg leaves the floor. Keep the elbows straight and shoulders stabilised.

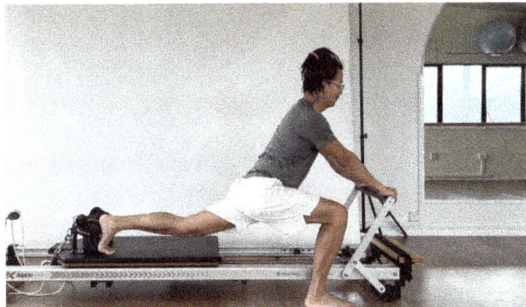

C
INHALE

1. Return to position **A**.
2. Repeat on the other side.

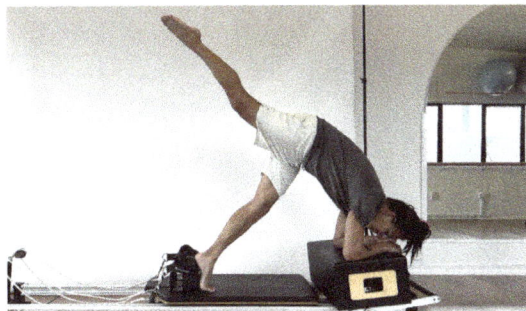

MODIFICATION

1. Forearms on top of the box.

THREE TOED SLOTH III

Strength: Chest, shoulders, arms, abs, quads, glutes, hamstrings

Level: Advanced   **Repetition:** 8-10   **Springs:** Medium to light

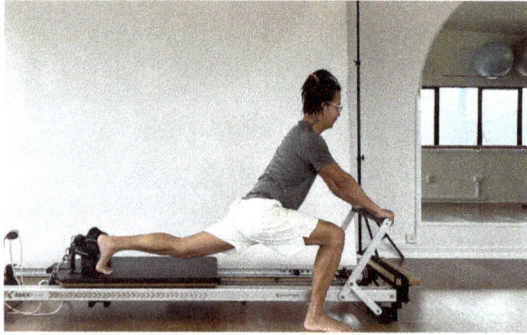

A
START

1. Scooter position, hands on the footbar.
2. Place your outer leg on the floor below your shoulder. Bend the knee as you extend the inner leg.
3. The inner leg extends behind you with your toes tucked under against the shoulder rest.

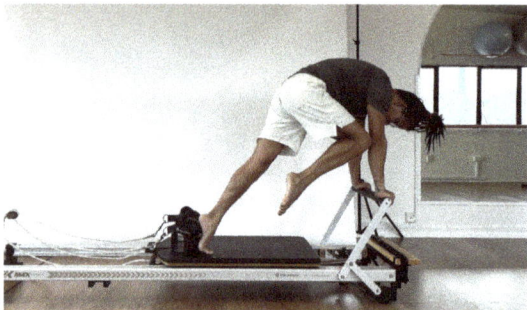

B
EXHALE

1. Pike up bringing your outer knee forward to the outside of your elbow on the same side as your leg leaves the floor.
2. Your spine curves.
3. The carriage closes.

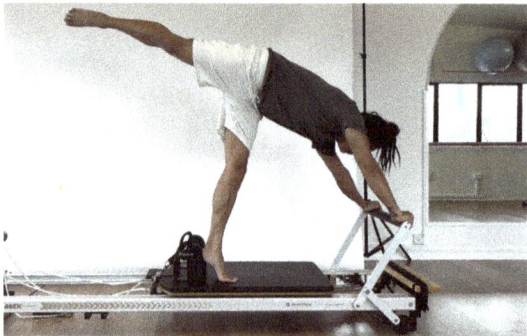

C
INHALE

1. Extend the outer leg behind you, straightening the knee. Your spine extends to neutral.

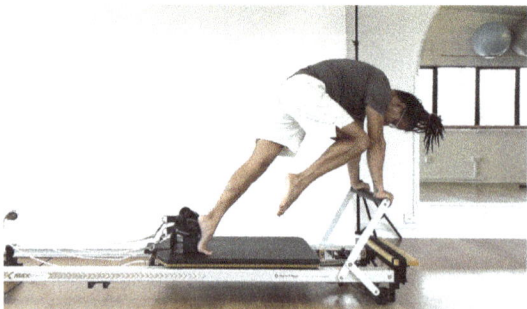

D
EXHALE

1. Return to position **B**.

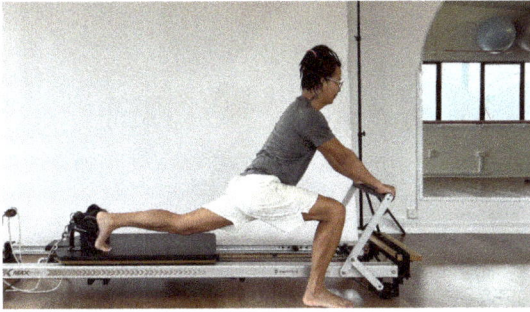

E

INHALE

1. Return to position **A**.
2. Repeat on the other side.

MODIFICATION

1. Forearms on top of the box.

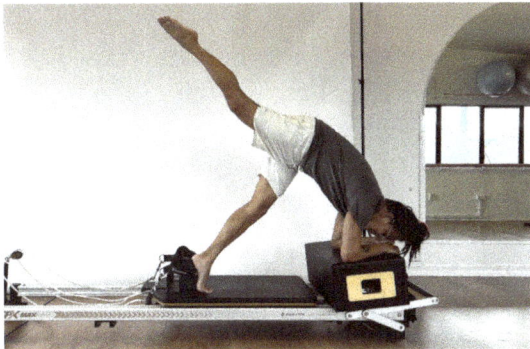

THREE TOED SLOTH IV

Strength: Chest, shoulders, arms, abs, quads, glutes, hamstrings

Level: Advanced   **Repetition:** 8-10   **Springs:** Medium to light

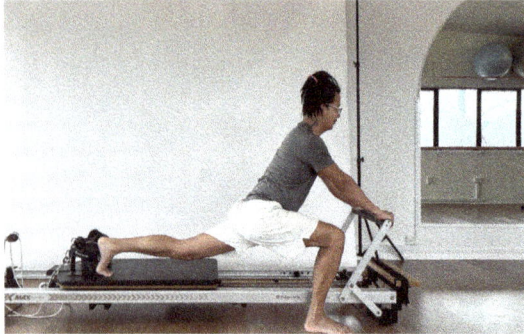

A
START

1. Scooter position, hands on the footbar
2. Place your outer leg on the floor below your shoulder. Bend the knee as you extend the inner leg.
3. The inner leg extends behind you with your toes tucked under against the shoulder rest.

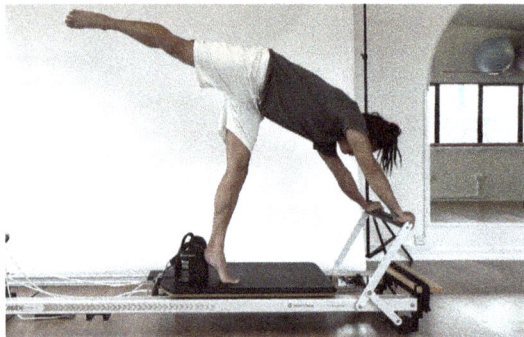

B
EXHALE

1. Pike up extending the outer leg behind you as you close the carriage.

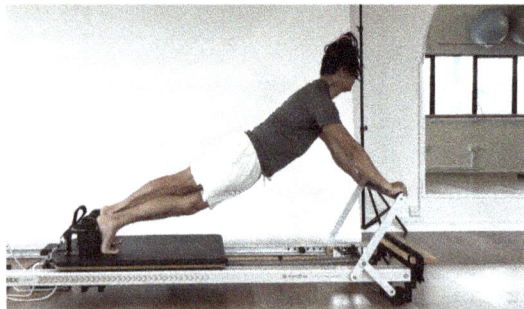

C
INHALE

1. Lower the leg and cross it underneath the other leg. Place your toes against the opposite shoulder pad.
2. Extend your spine slightly and gaze forward.

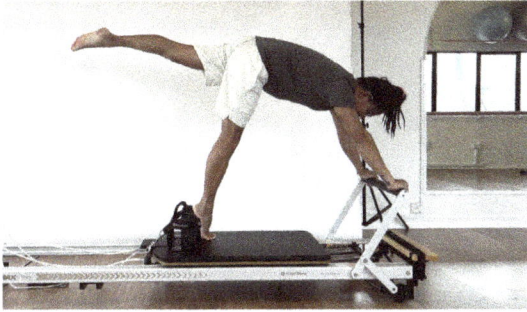

D

EXHALE

1. Extend the crossed leg back up behind you again as you close the carriage.

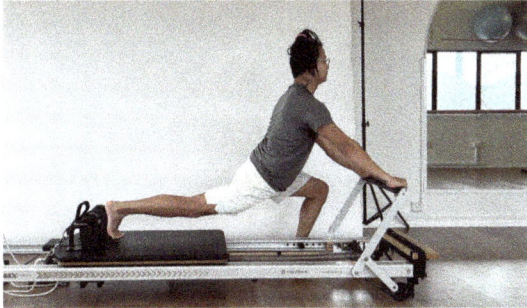

E

INHALE

1. Return to position **A**.
2. Repeat on the other side.

THE BLIND SIDE I

Strength: Shoulder, obliques, inner thighs

Level: Intermediate   **Repetition:** 8-10   **Springs:** Medium to light

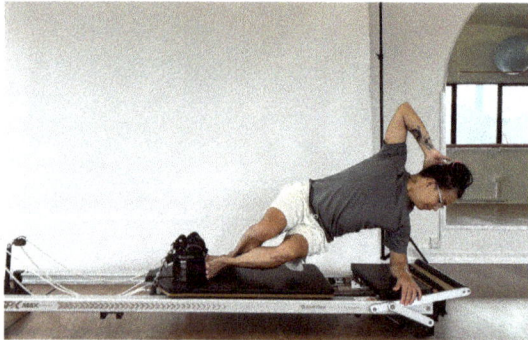

A
START

1. Side plank position with forearm on the standing platform.
2. Place the upper hand behind your head
3. Knees are bent with the lower foot placed against the front shoulder rest. The upper foot against the back shoulder rests.
4. Your hips are elevated off the carriage.

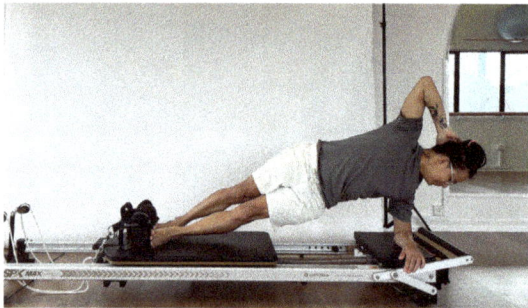

B
EXHALE

1. Push the carriage out straightening your legs. Push through your heels to engage your glutes more.

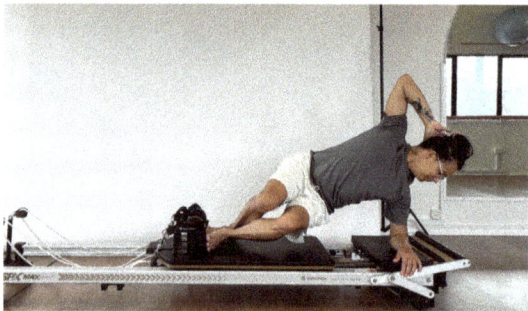

C
INHALE

1. Return to position **A**.
2. Repeat on the other side.

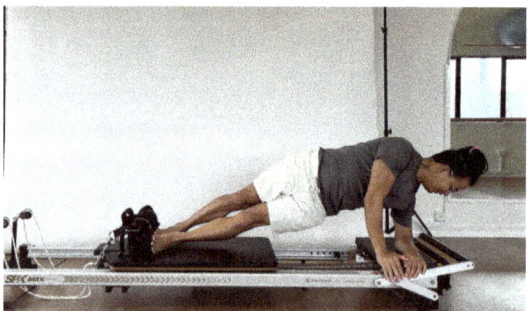

MODIFICATION

1. Place the top hand on the platform too.

PROGRESSION 1

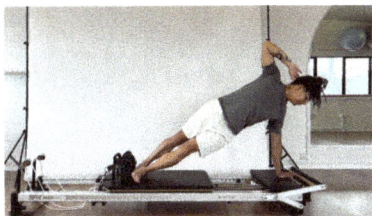

1. Extended arm with hand placed on the platform **(B)**

PROGRESSION 2

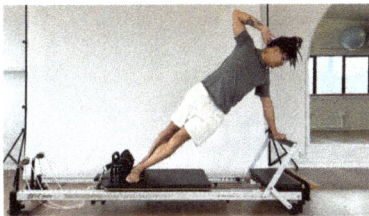

1. Hand on the footbar **(B)**

MODIFICATION

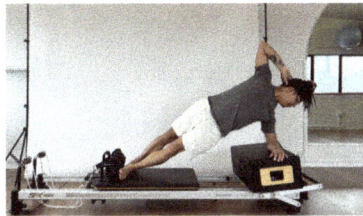

1. Forearm on top of the box **(B)**

THE BLIND SIDE II

Strength: Shoulder, obliques, inner thighs

Level: Intermediate   **Repetition:** 8-10   **Springs:** Medium to light

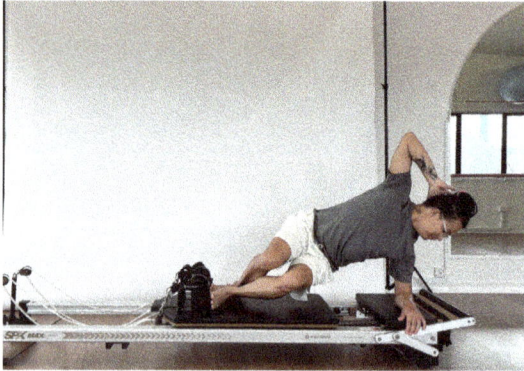

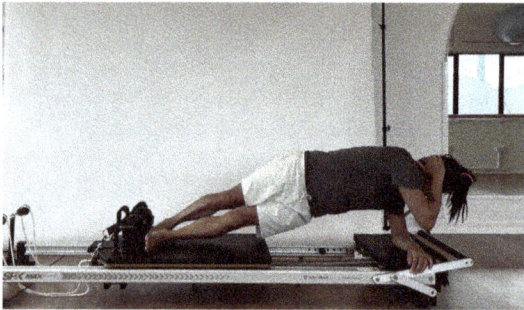

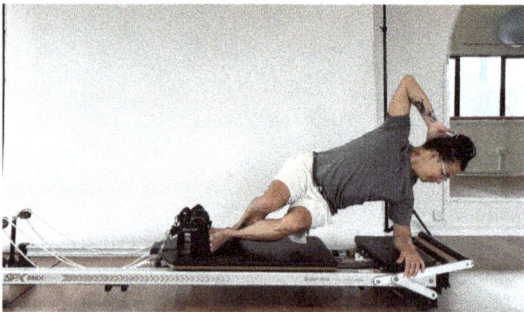

A
START

1. Side plank position with forearm on the standing platform.
2. Place the upper hand behind your head.
3. Knees are bent with the lower foot placed against the front shoulder rest. The upper foot against the back shoulder rest.
4. Your hips are elevated off the carriage.

B
EXHALE

1. Extend your legs keeping the heels down and twist your ribs.
2. Bring your upper elbow around to touch your lower hand.

C
INHALE

1. Return to position **A**.
2. Repeat on the other side.

PROGRESSION 1

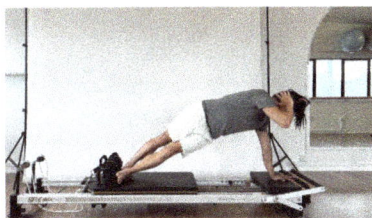

1. Extended arm with hand placed on the platform **(B)**

PROGRESSION 2

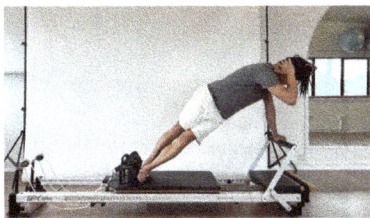

1. Hand on the footbar **(B)**

MODIFICATION

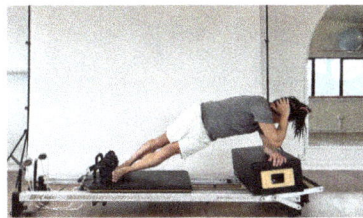

1. Forearm on top of the box **(B)**

RAINBOW I

Strength: Shoulder, obliques, inner thighs

Level: Advance   **Repetition:** 8-10   **Springs:** Medium to light

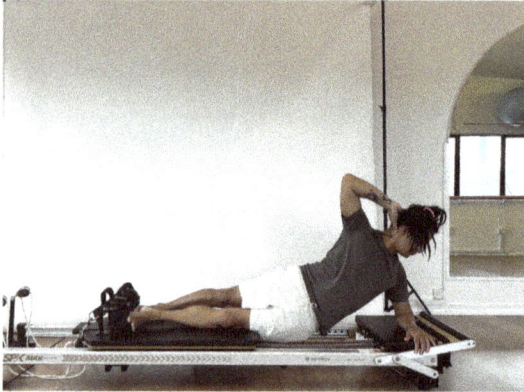

A
START

1. Side plank on your forearm with both legs extended. Place your top foot on the shoulder rest behind you. Place your lower foot on the front shoulder rest. Make sure you lower your heels pushing them backward.
2. Place your lower elbow on the standing platform.
3. Place your upper hand behind your head.

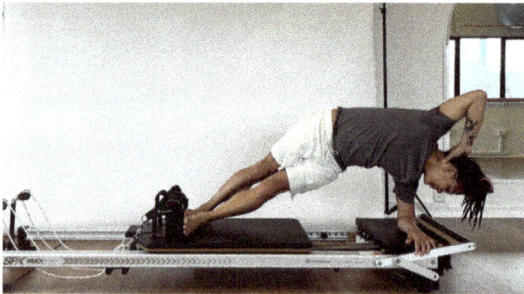

B
EXHALE

1. Lift your hips up to the ceiling, contracting your lower side into a side bend.

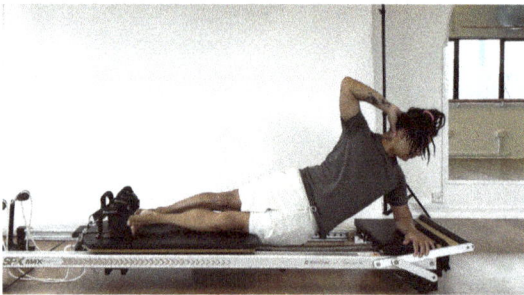

C
INHALE

1. Return to position **A**.
2. Repeat on the other side.

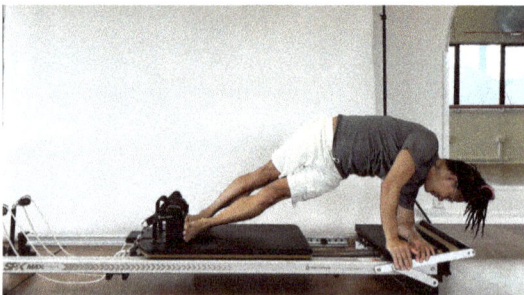

MODIFICATION

1. Place your top hand on the standing platform as well.

RAINBOW II

Strength: Shoulder, arms, obliques, inner thighs, glutes

Level: Advance   **Repetition:** 8-10   **Springs:** Medium to light

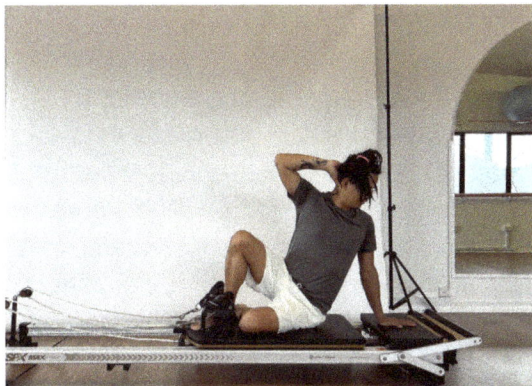

A
START

1. Sit on the carriage, facing sideways.
2. Bend your lower leg and place your foot against the back shoulder rest. Your front leg is bent, knee facing the ceiling. Your toes pressing against the front shoulder rest.
3. Place your hand on the standing platform with the elbow straight. Place the upper hand behind your head.

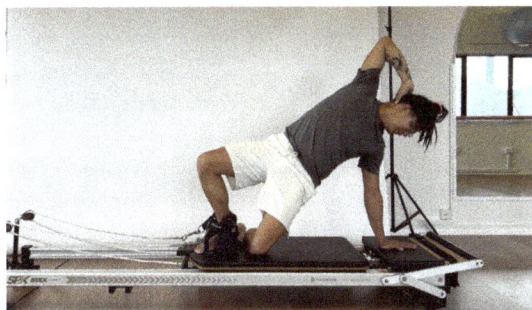

B
EXHALE

1. Lift your hips as you press your lower leg's shin into the carriage.
2. The carriage stays still.

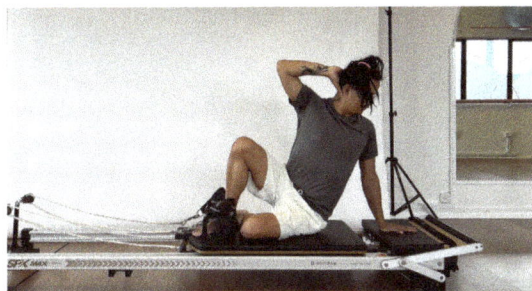

C
INHALE

1. Return to position **A**.
2. Repeat on the other side.

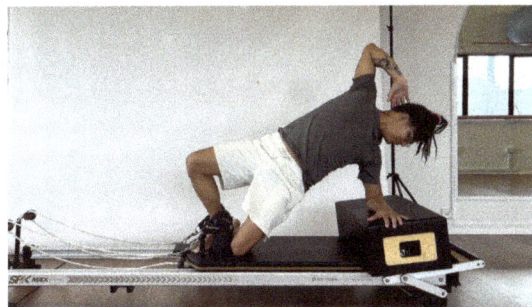

MODIFICATION

1. Forearm on top of the box.

RAINBOW III

Strength: Shoulders, arms, obliques, inner thighs, glutes

Level: Advanced   **Repetition:** 8-10   **Springs:** Medium to light

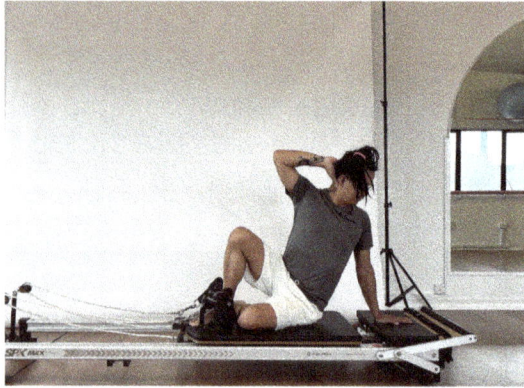

A
START

1. Sit on the carriage, facing sideways.
2. Bend your lower leg and place your foot against the back shoulder rest. Your front leg is bent, knee facing the ceiling. Your toes pressing against the front shoulder rest.
3. Place your hand on the standing platform with the elbow straight. Place the upper hand behind your head.

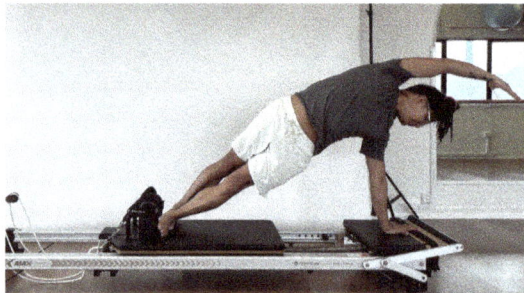

B
EXHALE

1. Lift your hips as you extend both legs opening the carriage.

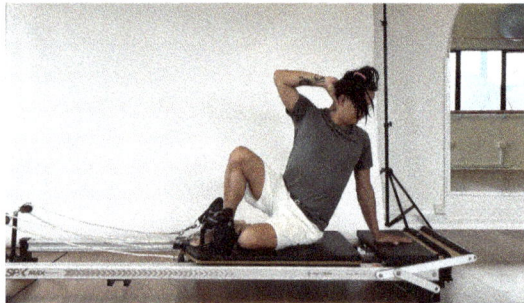

C
INHALE

1. Return to position **A**.
2. Repeat on the other side.

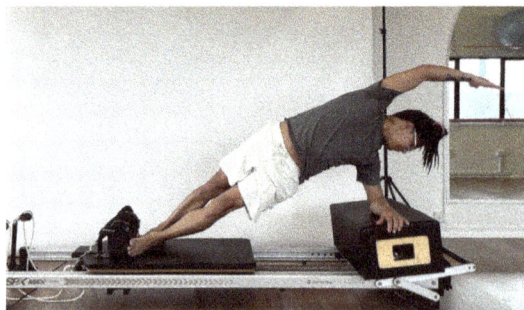

MODIFICATION

1. Forearm on top of the box.

ROLLER COASTER I

Strength: Chest, shoulders, arms, abs, quads, glutes

Level: Advanced   **Repetition:** 8-10   **Springs:** Medium to light

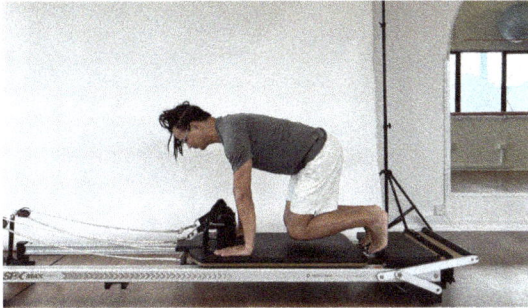

A
START

1. Neutral, four point kneeling position.
2. Place your hands beside shoulder rests.
3. Place your feet against the inner edge of the reformer frame or platform extender.
4. Lift your knees slightly off the carriage

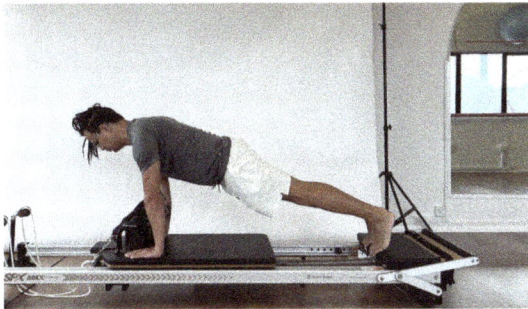

B
EXHALE

1. Extend your legs opening the carriage.

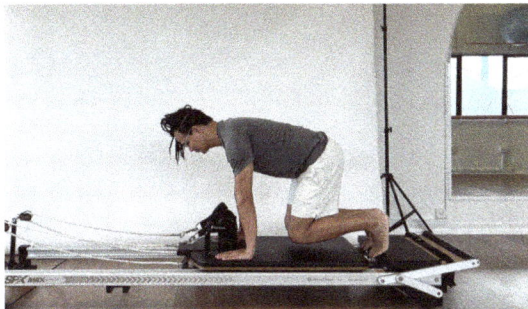

C
INHALE

1. Return to position **A**.

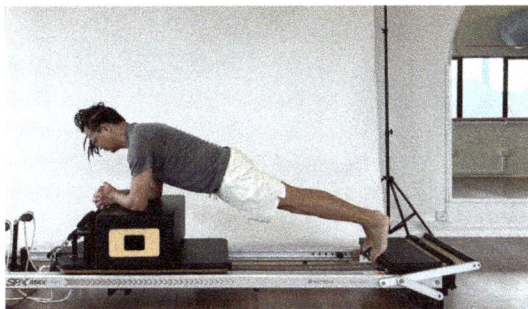

MODIFICATION

1. Place the box in front of the shoulder rests. Place your forearms on top of the box.

VARIATION

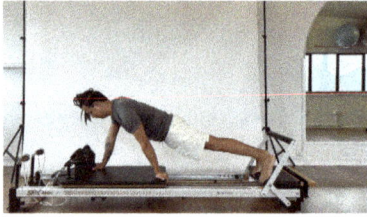

1. Place one hand at the front edge of the carriage **(B)**

PROGRESSION 1

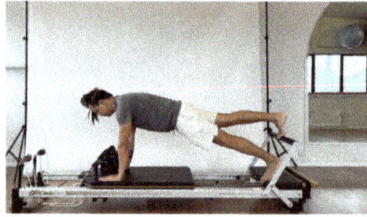

1. Place one foot on the footbar **(B)**

PROGRESSION 2

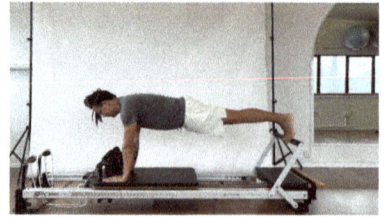

1. Both feet on footbar **(B)**

ROLLER COASTER II

Strength: Chest, shoulder, arms, abs, quads

Level: Advance   **Repetition:** 8-10   **Springs:** Medium to light

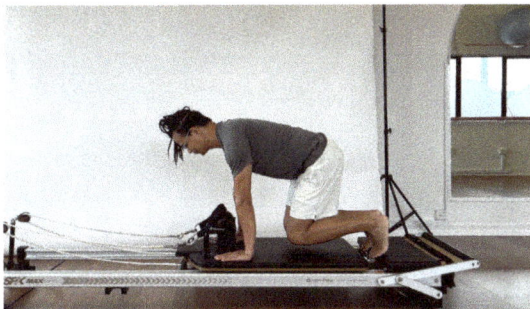

A
START

1. Neutral, four point kneeling position.
2. Place your hands beside shoulder rests.
3. Place your feet against the inner edge of the reformer frame or platform extender.
4. Lift your knees slightly off the carriage.

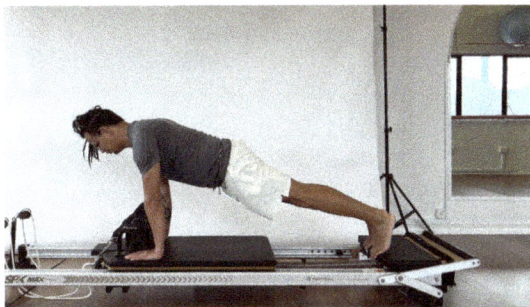

B
EXHALE

1. Extend both legs opening the carriage.

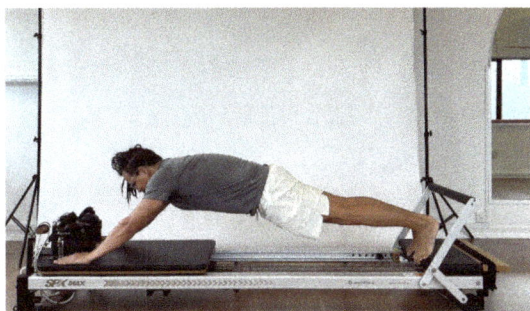

C
INHALE

1. Extend both arms moving the carriage out a little more.

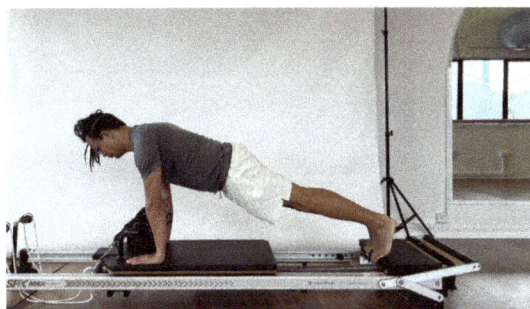

D
EXHALE

1. Return to position **B**.

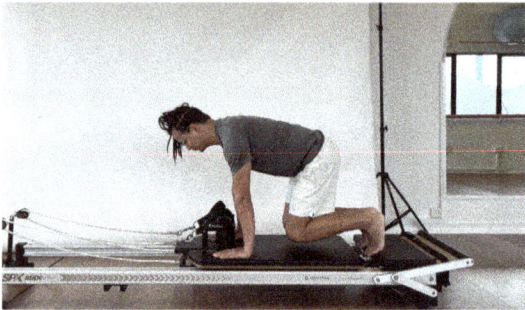

E

INHALE

1. Return to position **A**.

MODIFICATION

1. Place both elbows on top of the box.

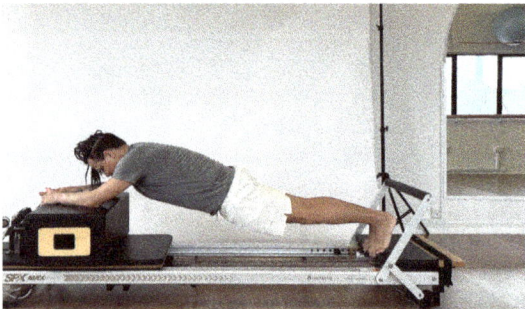

VARIATION

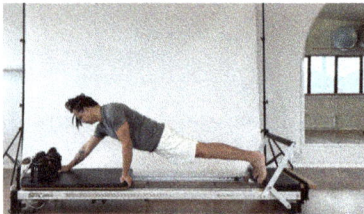

1. Place one hand on the front corner of the carriage **(C)**

PROGRESSION 1

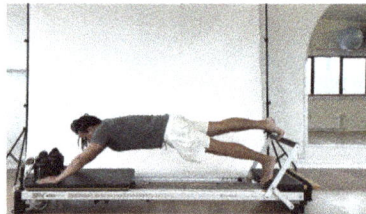

1. Place one foot on the footbar **(C)**

PROGRESSION 2

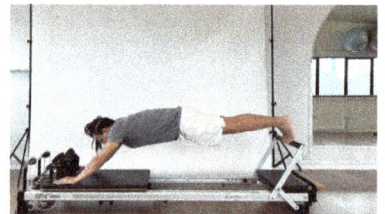

1. Place both feet on the footbar **(C)**

ROLLER COASTER III

Strength: Chest, shoulders, arms, abs, quads, glutes, hamstrings

Level: Advance   **Repetition:** 8-10   **Springs:** Medium to light

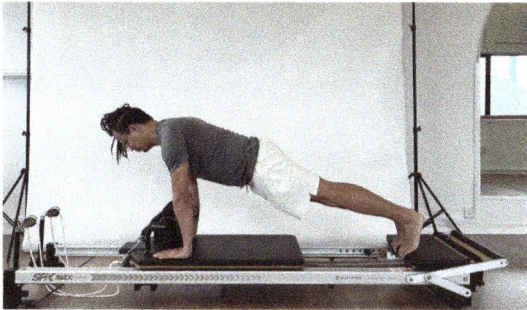

A
START

1. Neutral plank position.
2. Place both hands beside the shoulder rests.
3. Your feet press against the inside edge of the reformer frame or platform extender.

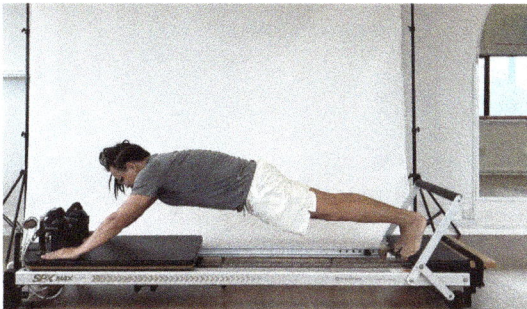

B
EXHALE

1. Push the carriage out with your arms.

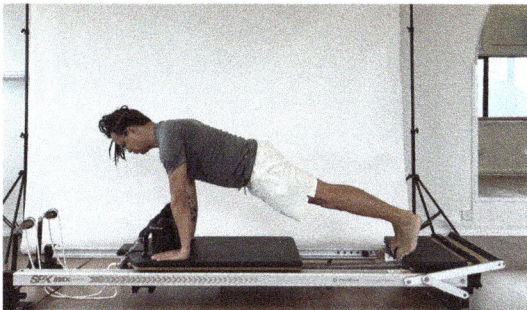

C
INHALE

1. Return to position **A**.

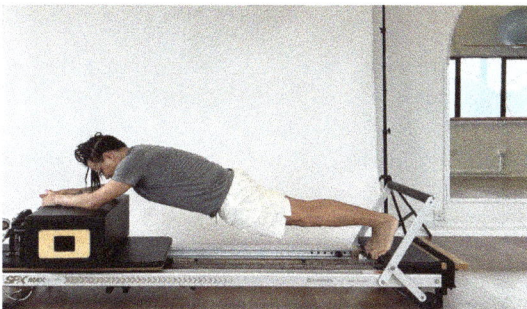

MODIFICATION

1. Place your elbows on top of the box.

VARIATION

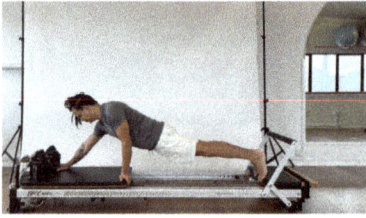

1. Place one hand on the front corner of the carriage **(B)**

PROGRESSION 1

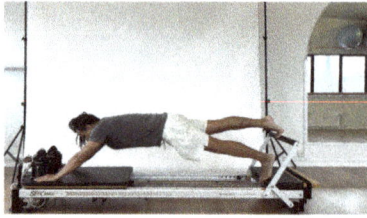

1. Place one foot on the footbar **(B)**

PROGRESSION 2

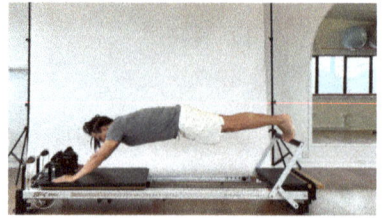

1. Place both feet on the footbar **(B)**

ROLLER COASTER IV

Strength: Chest, shoulders, arms, abs, quads, glutes and hamstrings

Level: Advanced   **Repetition:** 8-10   **Springs:** Medium to light

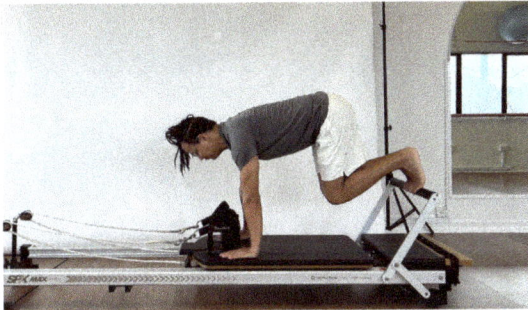

A
START

1. Place both hands beside shoulder rests and the balls of your feet on the footbar.
2. Both knees are bent in an elevated four point kneeling position.
3. Your spine is in a neutral position.

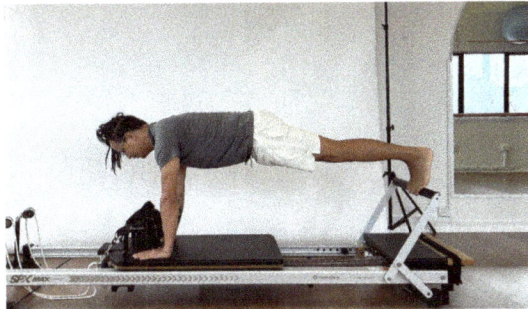

B
EXHALE

1. Straighten your legs and push the carriage out.

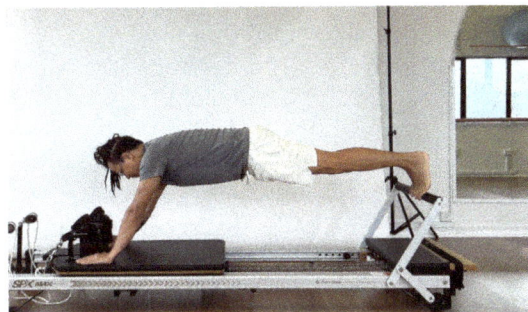

C
INHALE

1. Extend your arms a little further forward.

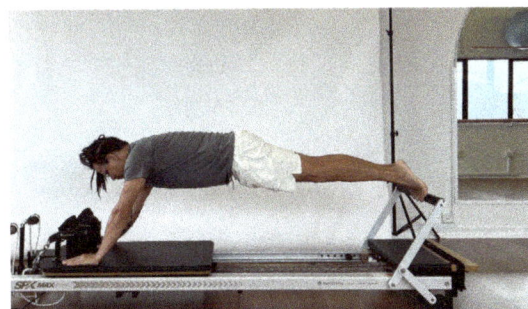

D
EXHALE

1. Lift your heels as if doing a calf raise.

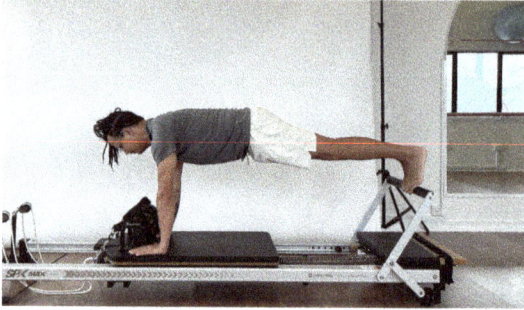

E

INHALE

1. Return to position **B**.

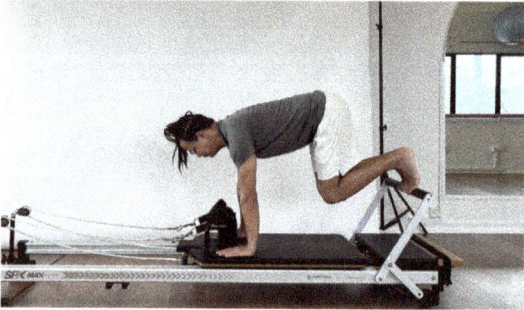

F

EXHALE

1. Return to position **A**.

BOOSTER I

Strength: Chest, shoulders, arms, abs, quads, glutes and hamstrings

Level: Advanced   **Repetition:** 8-10   **Springs:** Medium to light

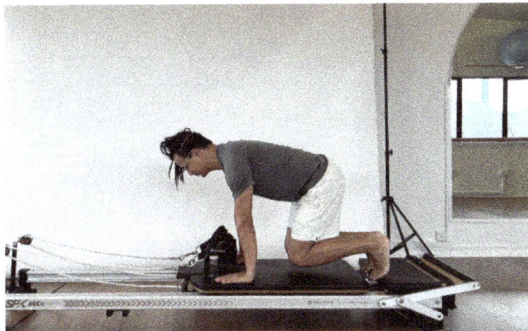

A
START

1. Neutral four point kneeling position with your toes tucked and pressing against the reformer frame or standing platform extender.
2. Place your hands beside the shoulder rests.
3. Float your knees a couple of centimeters off the carriage.

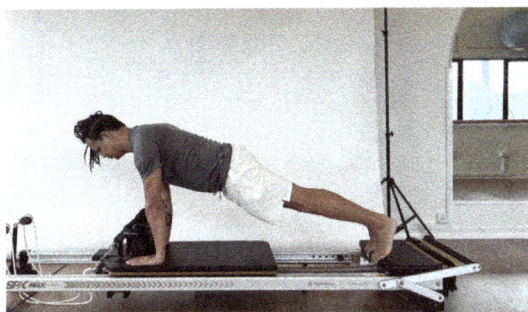

B
EXHALE

1. Extend your legs pushing the carriage forward.

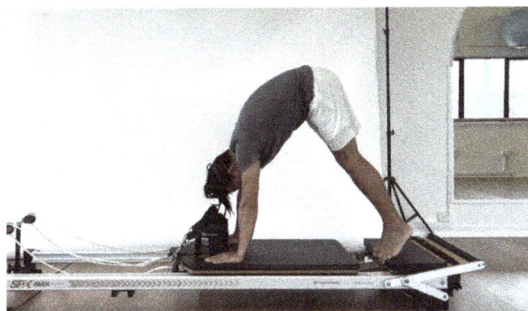

C
INHALE

1. Lift your hips to the ceiling, drawing the carriage in toward the footbar.

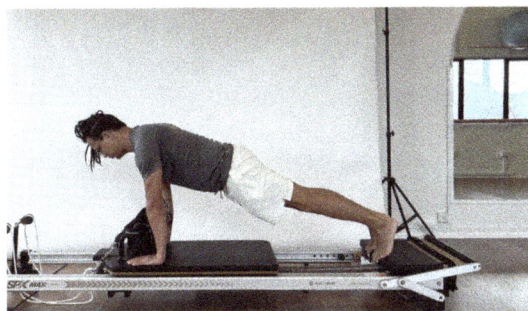

D
EXHALE

1. Return to position **B**.

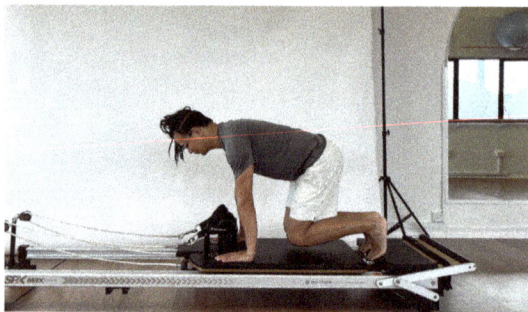

E

INHALE

1. Return to position **A**.

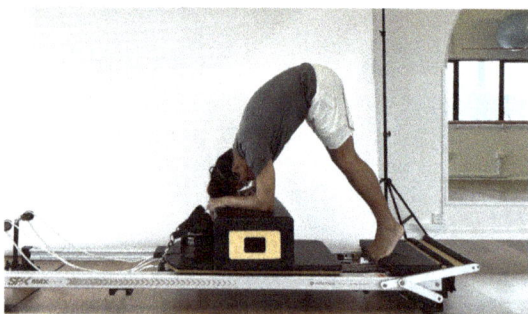

MODIFICATION

1. Place both elbows on top of the box.

VARIATION

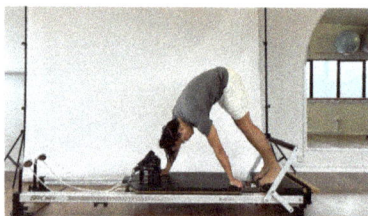

1. Place one hand on the front corner of the carriage **(C)**

PROGRESSION 1

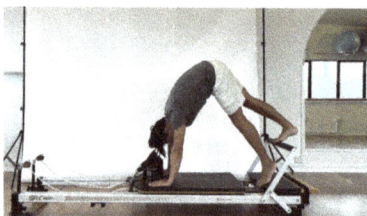

1. Place one foot on the footbar **(C)**

PROGRESSION 2

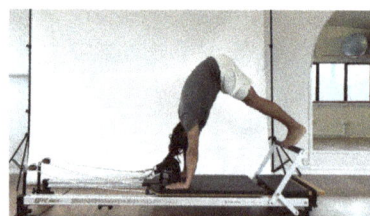

1. Place both feet on the footbar **(C)**

PROGRESSION 3

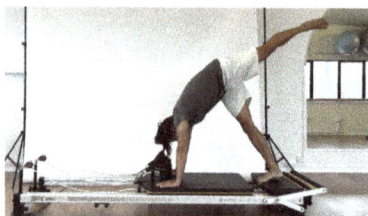

1. Place one foot on the standing platform and extend the other leg up to the ceiling **(C)**

PROGRESSION 4

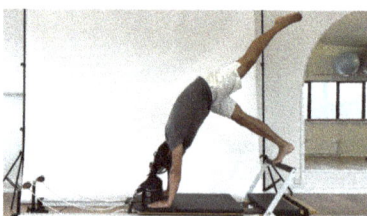

1. Place one foot on the footbar and extend the other up toward the ceiling **(C)**

BOOSTER II

Strength: Chest, shoulder, arms, abs, quads, glutes, and hamstrings

Level: Advance   **Repetition:** 8-10   **Springs:** Medium to light

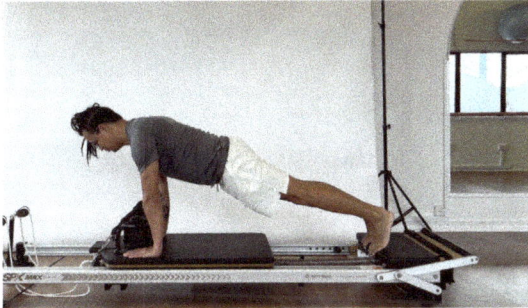

A
START

1. Neutral plank position with your toes tucked and pressing against the reformer frame or standing platform extender.
2. Place your hands beside the shoulder rests.

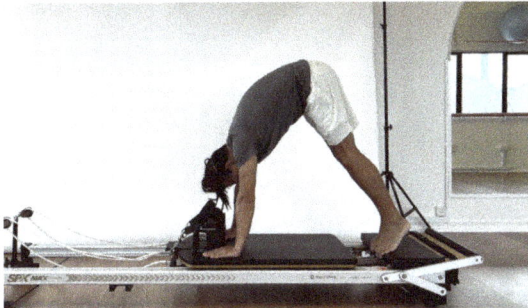

B
EXHALE

1. Lift your hips up to the ceiling, closing the carriage.

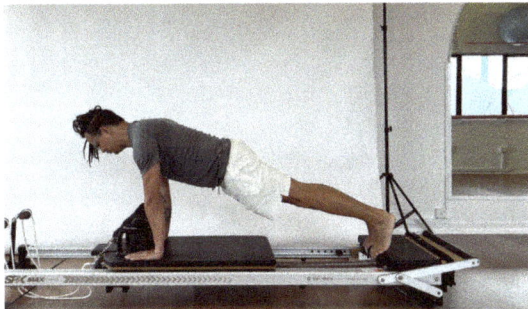

C
INHALE

1. Return to position **A**.

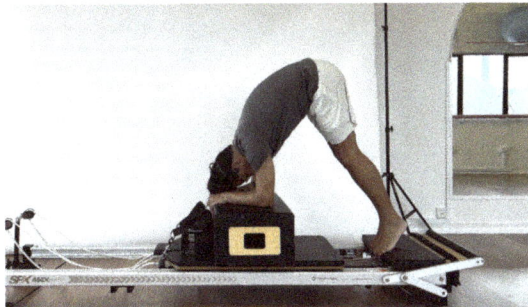

MODIFICATION

1. Place your forearms on top of the reformer box.

VARIATION

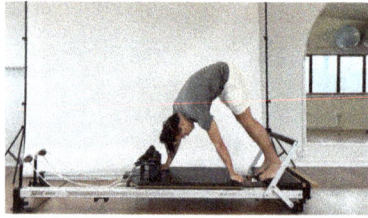

1. Place one hand on the front corner of the reformer carriage **(C)**

PROGRESSION 1

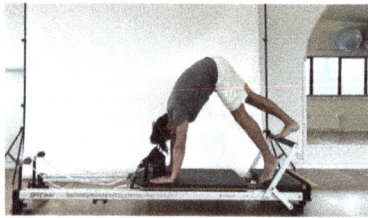

1. Place one foot on the footbar **(C)**

PROGRESSION 2

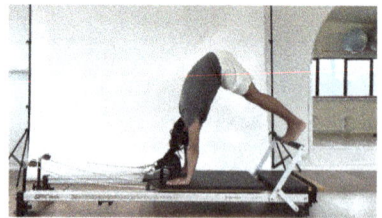

1. Place both feet on the footbar **(C)**

PROGRESSION 3

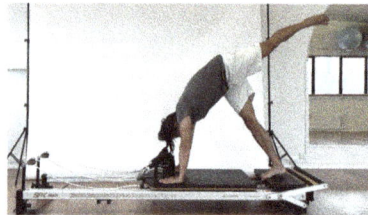

1. Place one foot on the standing platform **(C)**

PROGRESSION 4

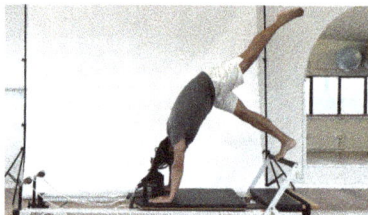

1. Place one foot on the footbar **(C)**

DRAGON'S TAIL I

Strength: Chest, shoulder, arms, abs, quads, glutes and hamstrings

Level: Advance   **Repetition:** 8-10   **Springs:** Medium to light

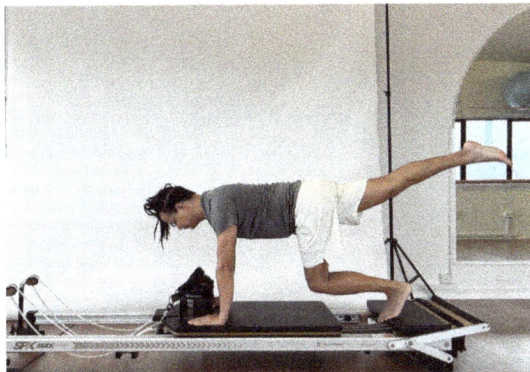

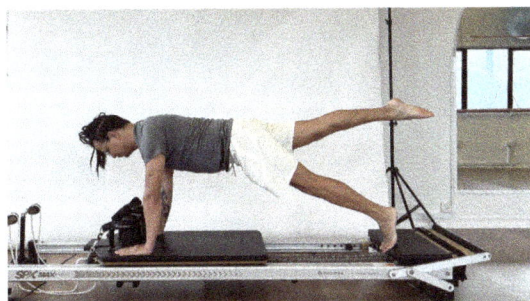

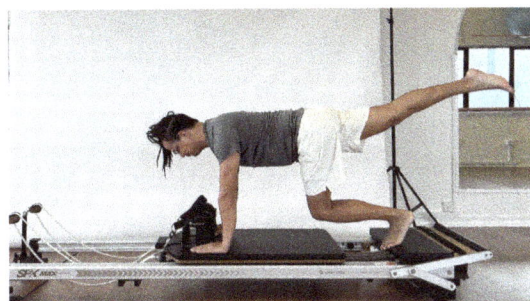

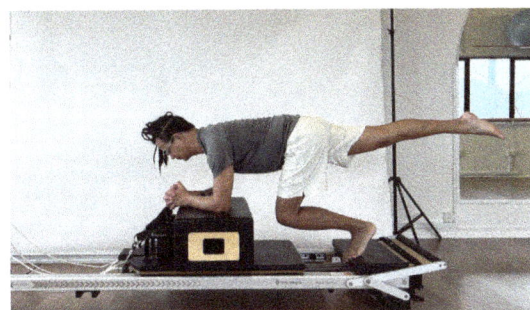

A

START

1. Neutral four point kneeling position with the toes of one foot tucked and pressing against the reformer frame or standing platform extender.
2. Extend the other leg out behind you parallel to the floor and in line with your hip.
3. Place your hands beside the shoulder rests.
4. Float your bent knee off the carriage.

B

EXHALE

1. Push out straightening your knee.

C

INHALE

1. Return to position **A**.
2. Repeat to the other side.

MODIFICATION

1. Place your forearms on top of the reformer box.

DRAGON'S TAIL II

Strength: Chest, shoulders, arms, abs, quads, glutes and hamstrings

Level: Advance   **Repetition:** 8-10   **Springs:** Medium to light

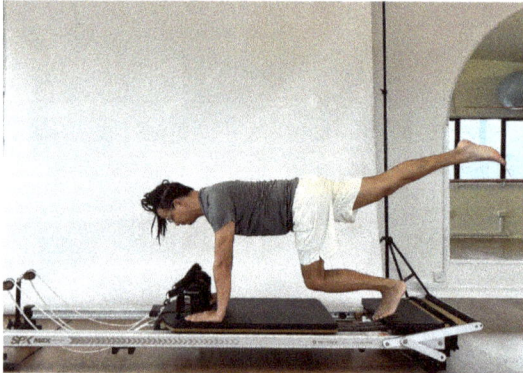

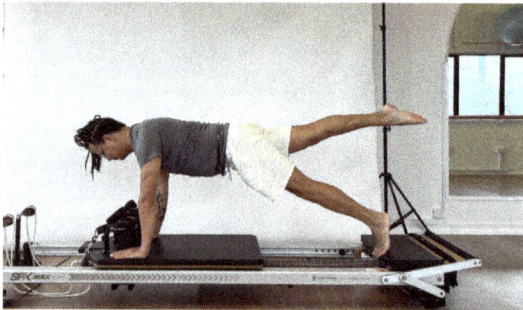

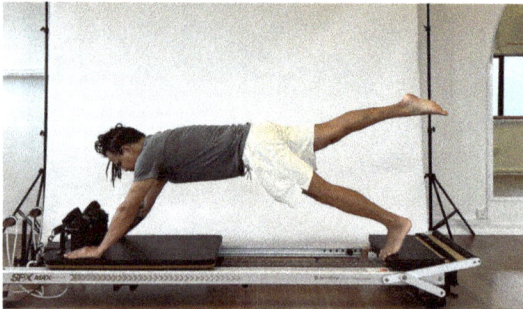

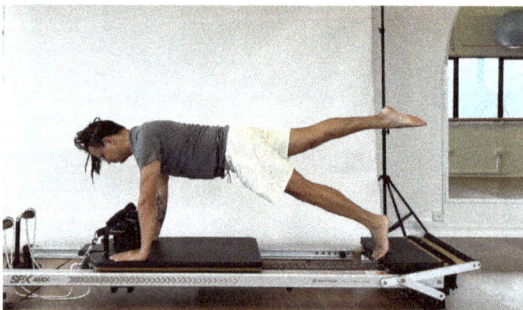

A
START

1. Neutral four point kneeling position with the toes of one foot tucked and pressing against the reformer frame or standing platform extender.
2. Extend the other leg out behind you parallel to the floor and in line with your hip.
3. Place your hands beside the shoulder rests.
4. Float your bent knee off the carriage.

B
EXHALE

1. Extend your leg opening the carriage.

C
INHALE

1. Push the carriage out a little further from your arms.

D
EXHALE

1. Return to position **B**.

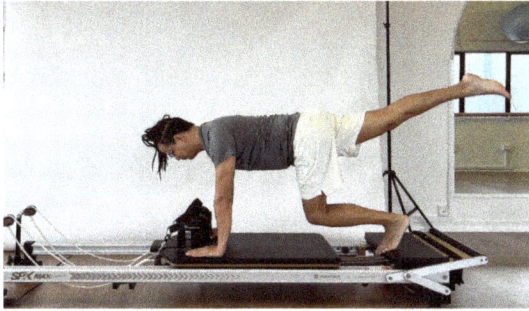

E

INHALE

1. Return to the starting position

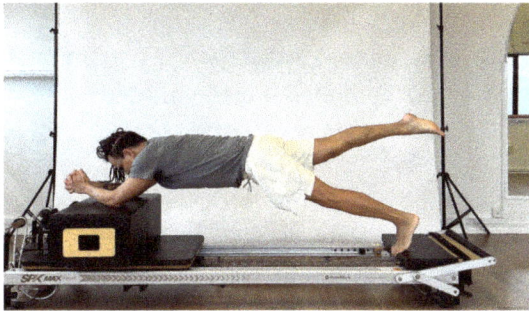

MODIFICATION

1. Place your elbows on top of the reformer box.

DRAGON'S TAIL III

Strength: Chest, shoulder, arms, abs, quads, glutes and hamstrings

Level: Advanced   **Repetition:** 8-10   **Springs:** Medium to light

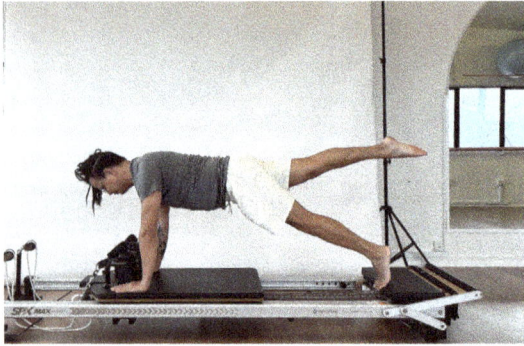

A
START

1. Neutral plank position with the toes of one foot tucked and pressing against the reformer frame or standing platform extender.
2. Extend the other leg out behind you parallel to the floor and in line with your hip.
3. Place your hands beside the shoulder rests.

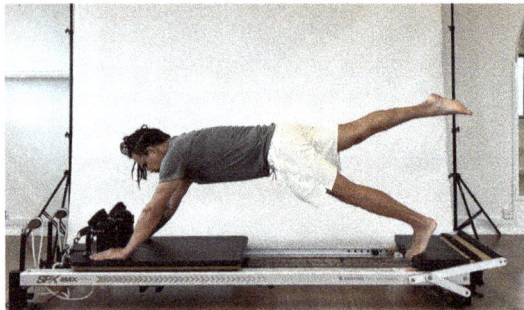

B
EXHALE

1. Extend your arms further forward, opening the carriage a little more.

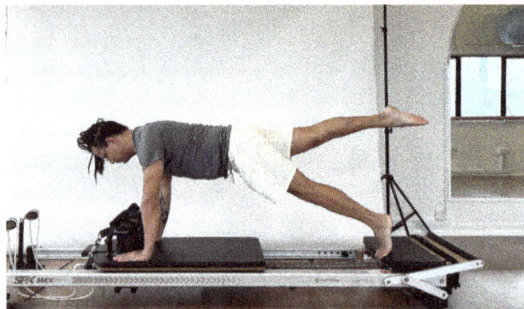

C
INHALE

1. Return to position **A**.
2. Repeat to the other side.

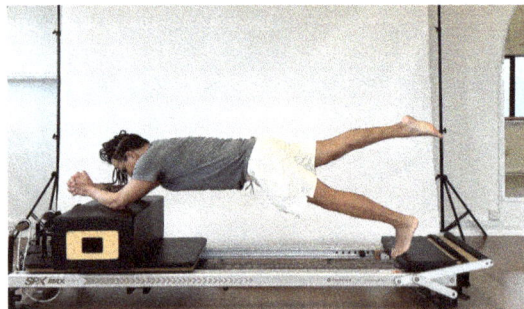

MODIFICATION

1. Place your elbows on top of the box.

DRAGON'S TAIL IV

Strength: Chest, shoulder, arms, abs, quads, glutes and hamstrings

Level: Advanced   **Repetition:** 8-10   **Springs:** Medium to light

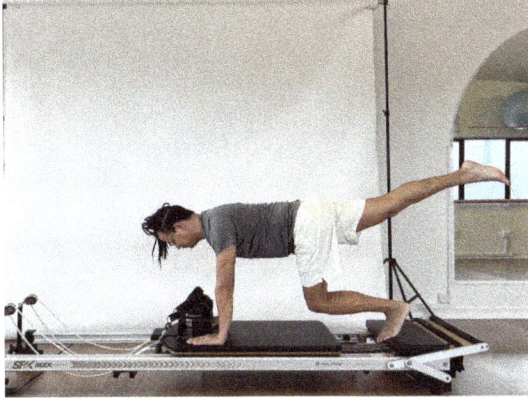

A
START

1. Neutral four point kneeling position with the toes of one foot tucked and pressing against the reformer frame or standing platform extender.
2. Extend the other leg out behind you parallel to the floor and in line with your hip.
3. Place your hands beside the shoulder rests.
4. Float your bent knee off the carriage.

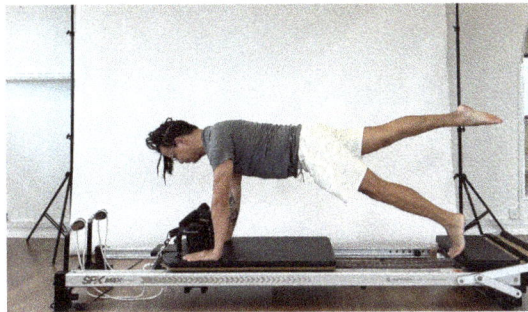

B
EXHALE

1. Extend your leg pushing the carriage out.

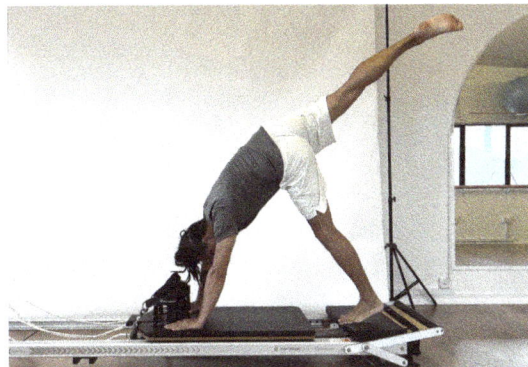

C
INHALE

1. Lift your hips and leg up to the ceiling, bringing the carriage into the closed position.

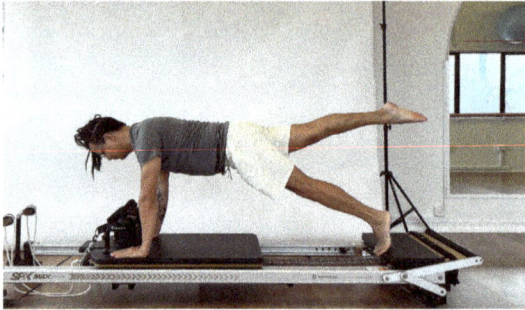

D
EXHALE

1. Return to position **B**.

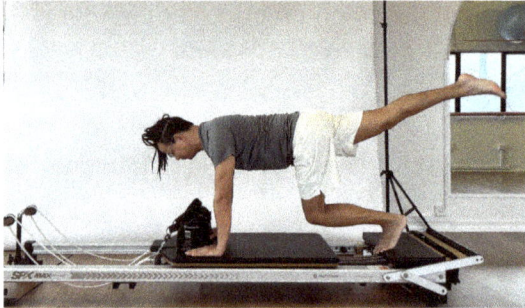

E
INHALE

1. Return to position **A**.
2. Repeat to the other side.

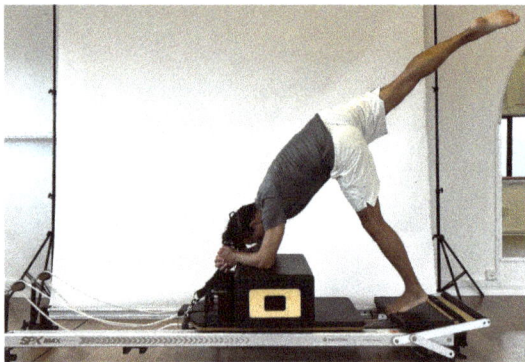

MODIFICATION

1. Place your elbows on top of the box.

DRAGON'S TAIL V

Strength: Chest, shoulders, arms, abs, quads, glutes and hamstrings

Level: Advance   **Repetition:** 8-10   **Springs:** Medium to light

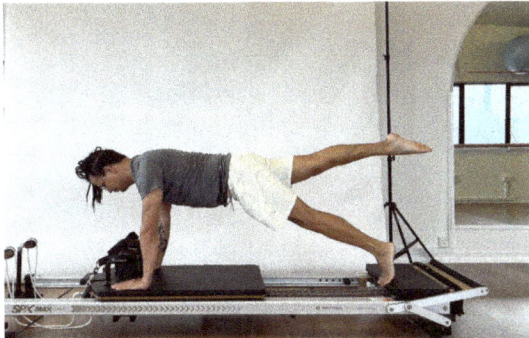

A
START

1. Neutral plank position with the toes of one foot tucked and pressing against the reformer frame or standing platform extender.
2. Extend the other leg out behind you parallel to the floor and in line with your hip.
3. Place your hands beside the shoulder rests.

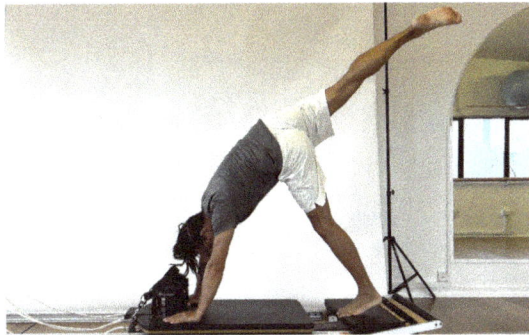

B
EXHALE

1. Lift your leg and hips up to the ceiling.

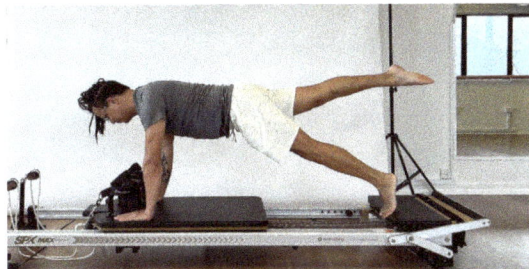

C
INHALE

1. Return to position **A**.

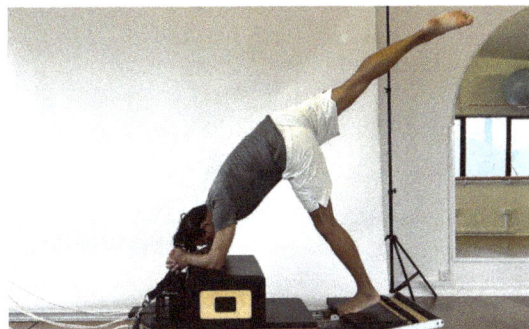

MODIFICATION

1. Place both elbows on top of the box.

BULLET TRAIN I

Strength: Chest, shoulders, abs, quads, glutes and hamstrings

Level: Intermediate   **Repetition:** 8-10   **Springs:** Medium to light

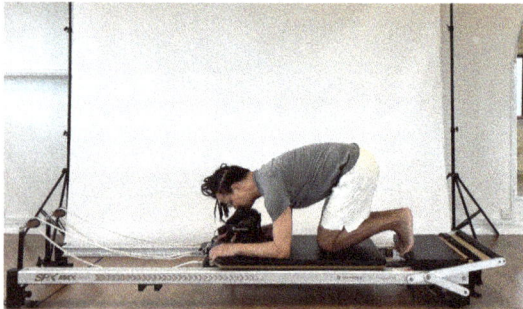

A
START

1. Neutral four point kneeling position. Place the forearms next to the shoulder rests.
2. Knees float off the carriage.
3. Place the feet on the inside edge of the reformer frame or standing platform.

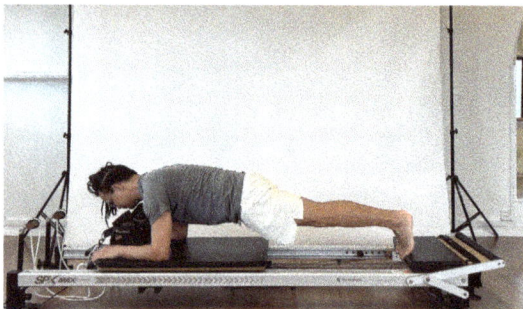

B
EXHALE

1. Extend your legs.

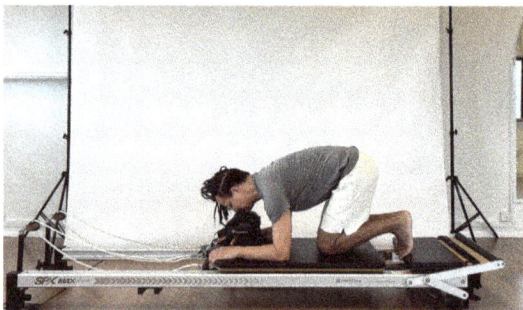

C
INHALE

1. Return to position **A**.

VARIATION

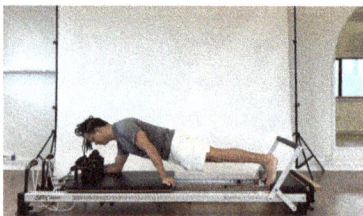

1. Place one hand on the front of the carriage **(B)**

PROGRESSION 1

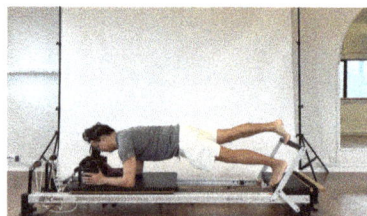

1. Place one foot on the footbar **(B)**

PROGRESSION 2

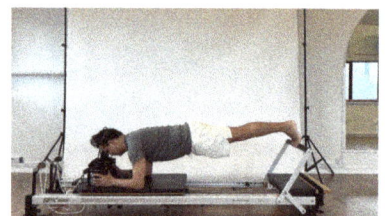

1. Place both feet on the footbar **(B)**

BULLET TRAIN II

Strength: Chest, shoulders, abs, quads, glutes and hamstrings

Level: Intermediate   **Repetition:** 8-10   **Springs:** Medium to light

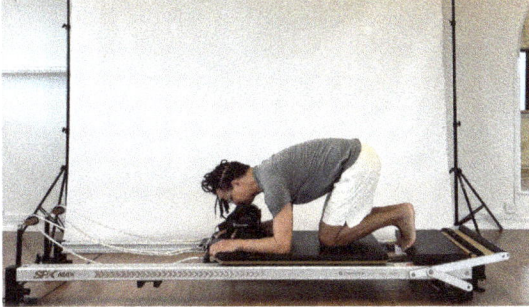

A
START

1. Neutral four point kneeling position. Place the forearms next to the shoulder rests.
2. Knees float off the carriage.
3. Place the feet on the inside edge of the reformer frame or standing platform.

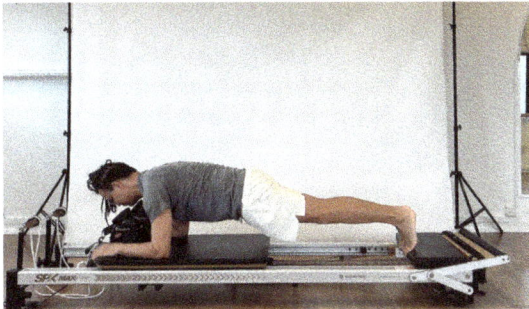

B
EXHALE

1. Extend your legs.

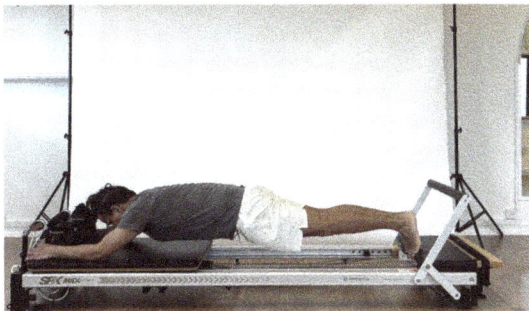

C
INHALE

1. Extend the carriage out further from your shoulders and arms.

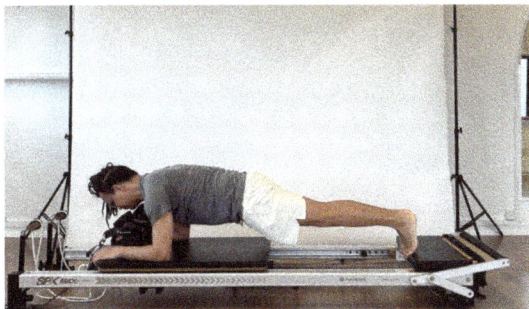

D
EXHALE

1. Return to position **B**.

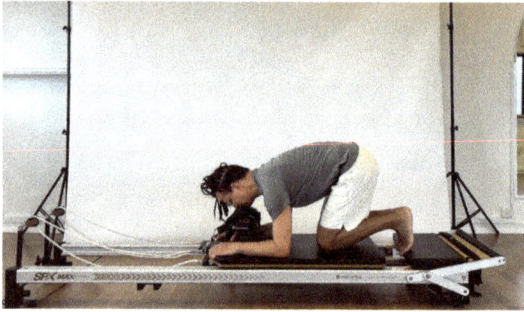

E

INHALE

1. Return to position **A**.

VARIATION

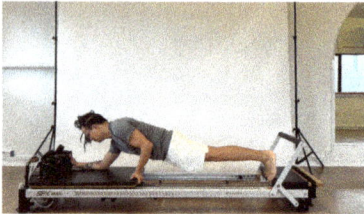

1. Place one hand at the front of carriage **(C)**

PROGRESSION 1

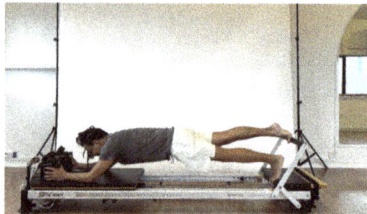

1. Place one foot on the footbar **(C)**

PROGRESSION 2

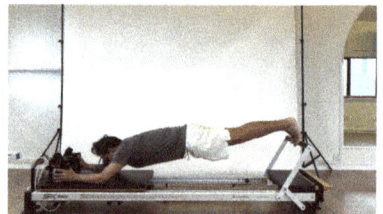

1. Place both feet on the footbar **(C)**

BULLET TRAIN III

Strength: Chest, shoulder, abs, quads

Level: Intermediate   **Repetition:** 8-10   **Springs:** medium to light

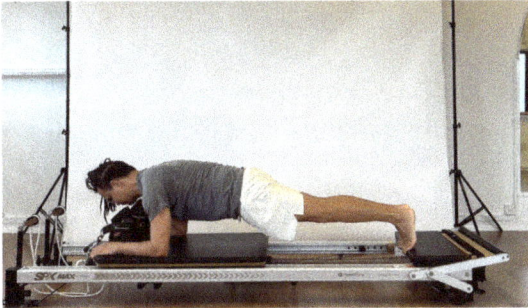

A
START

1. Neutral plank position on your forearms. Place the forearms next to the shoulder rests.
2. Place the feet on the inside edge of the reformer frame or standing platform.

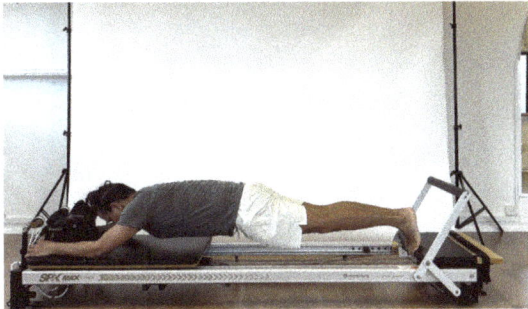

B
EXHALE

1. Push the carriage out further from your shoulders and arms.

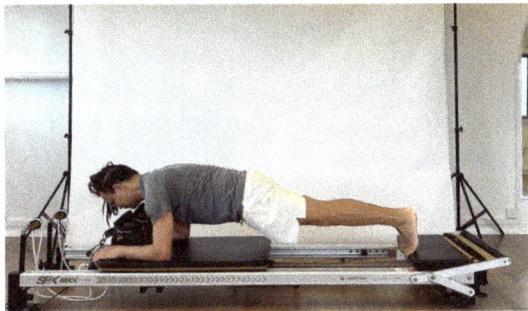

C
INHALE

1. Return to position **A**.

VARIATION

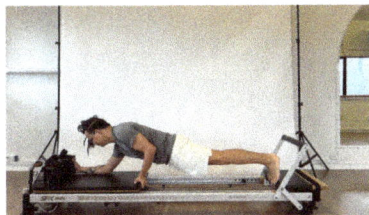

1. Place one hand at the front of carriage **(B)**

PROGRESSION 1

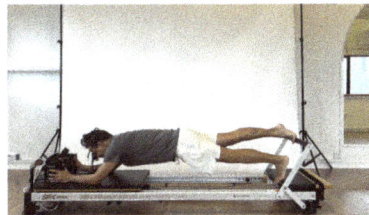

1. Place one foot on the footbar **(B)**

PROGRESSION 2

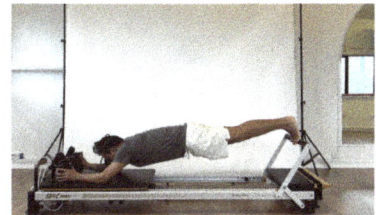

1. Place both feet on the footbar **(B)**

BULLET TRAIN IV

Strength: Chest, shoulders, abs, quads, glutes and hamstrings

Level: Advanced   **Repetition:** 8-10   **Springs:** Medium to light

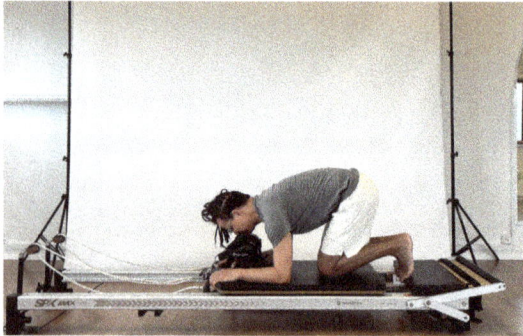

A
START

1. Neutral four point kneeling position. Place the forearms next to the shoulder rests.
2. Knees float off the carriage.
3. Place the feet on the inside edge of the reformer frame or standing platform.

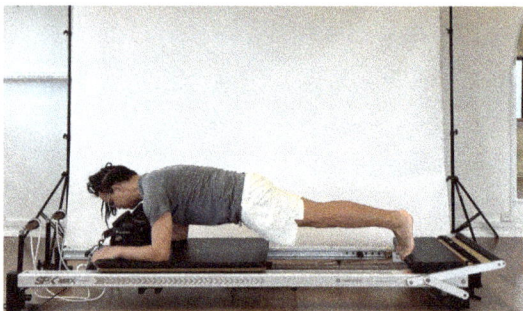

B
EXHALE

1. Extend both legs.

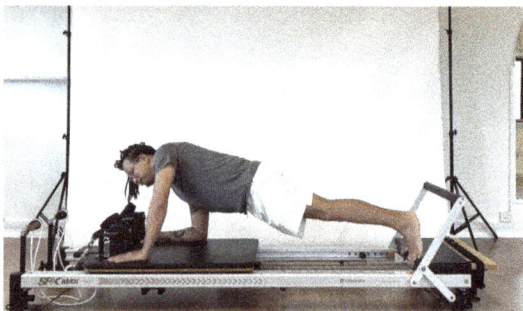

C
INHALE

1. Straighten one arm bringing the weight onto your hand.

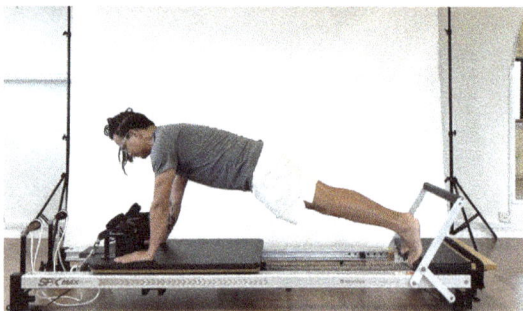

D
EXHALE

1. Extend the other arm.

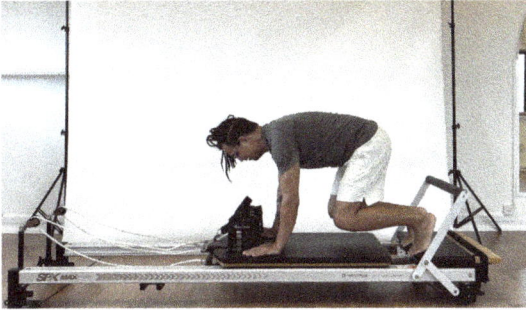

E

INHALE

1. Bend your knees and return the carriage.

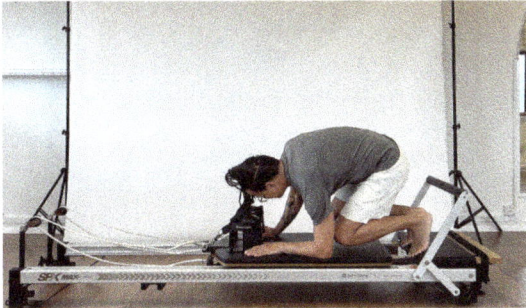

F

EXHALE

1. Lower one elbow down.

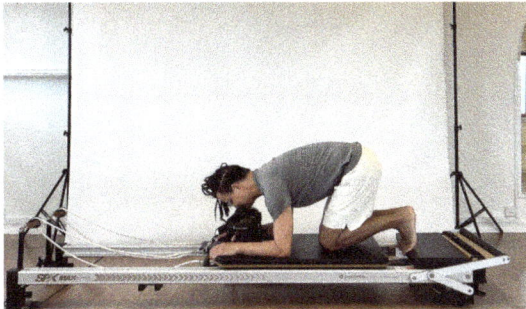

G

INHALE

1. Return to position **A**.

PROGRESSION 1

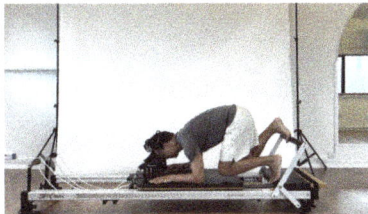

1. Place one foot on the footbar **(A)**

PROGRESSION 2

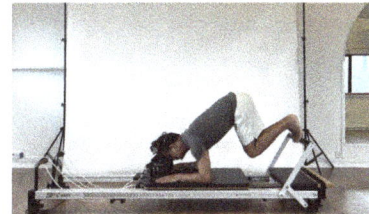

1. Place both feet on the footbar **(A)**

PYRAMID I

Strength: Chest, shoulders, abs, quads, glutes and hamstrings

Level: Advanced   **Repetition:** 8-10   **Springs:** Medium to light

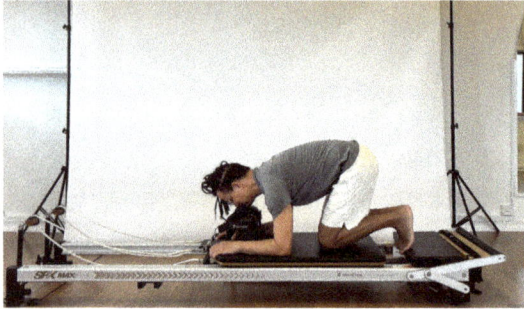

A
START

1. Neutral four point kneeling position. Place the forearms next to the shoulder rests.
2. Knees float off the carriage.
3. Place the feet on the inside edge of the reformer frame or standing platform.

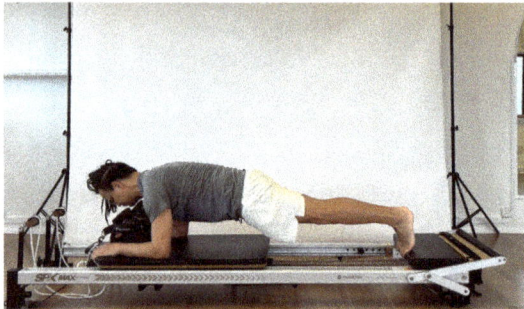

B
EXHALE

1. Extend your legs.

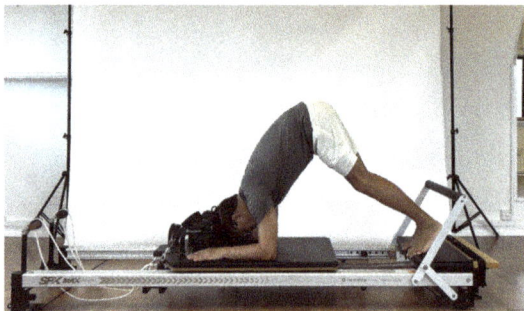

C
INHALE

1. Lift your hips up bringing the carriage toward the footbar.

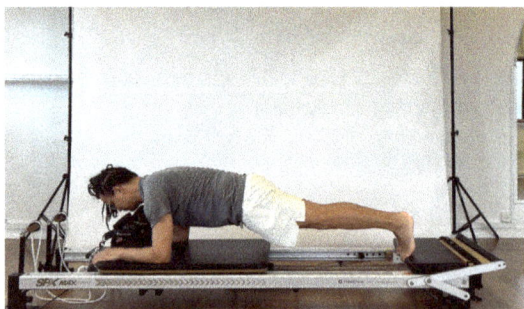

D
EXHALE

1. Return to position **B**.

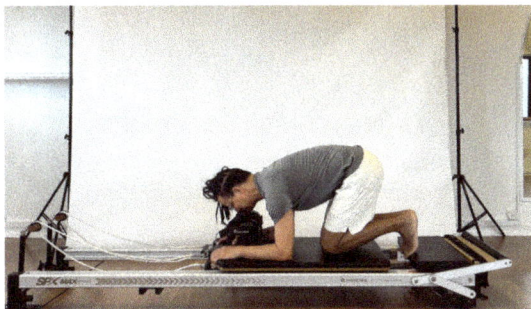

E
INHALE
1. Return to position **A**.

VARIATION

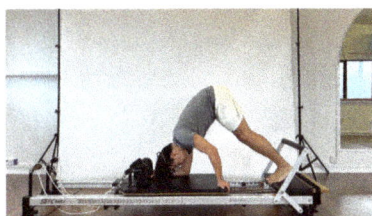

1. Place one hand on the front corner of the carriage **(C)**

PROGRESSION 1

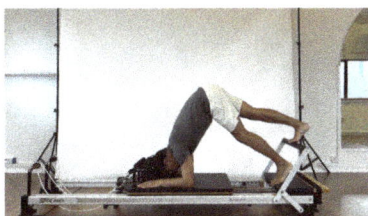

1. Place one foot on the footbar **(C)**

PROGRESSION 2

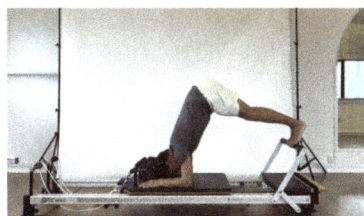

1. Place both feet on the footbar **(C)**

PROGRESSION 3

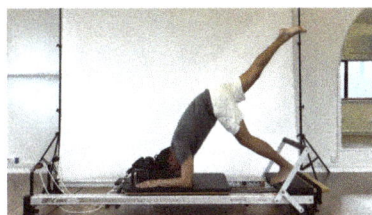

1. Extend one leg up toward the ceiling **(C)**

PROGRESSION 4

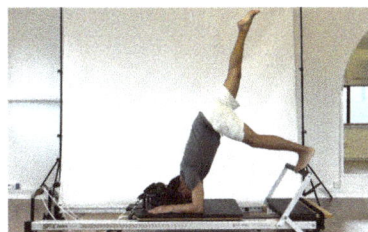

1. Place one foot on the footbar and extend the other leg up toward the ceiling **(C)**

PYRAMID II

Strength: Chest, shoulders, abs, quads

Level: Advanced   **Repetition:** 8-10   **Springs:** Medium to light

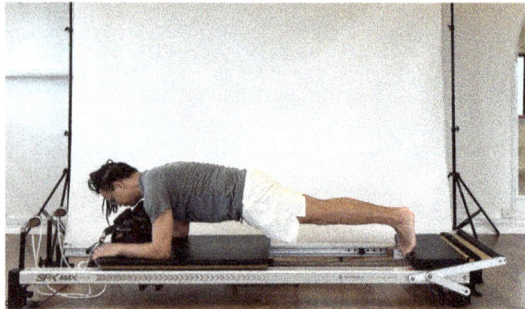

A
START

1. Neutral and in plank position on your forearms facing the risers.
2. Wedge your feet against the inside of the frame or standing platform.

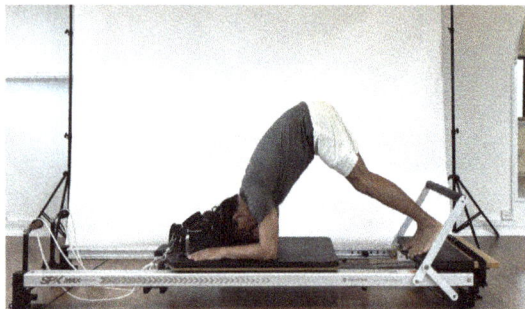

B
EXHALE

1. Lift your hips to the ceiling.

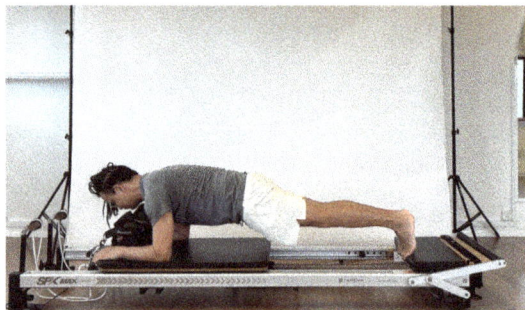

C
INHALE

1. Return to position **A**.

VARIATION

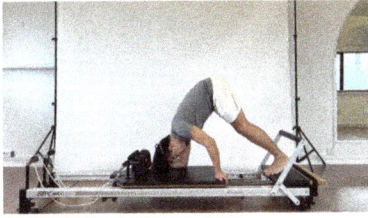

1. Place one hand on the front corner of the carriage **(C)**

PROGRESSION 1

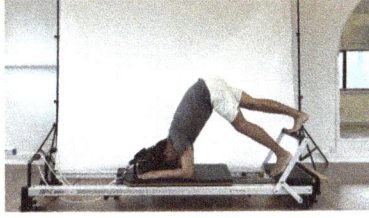

1. Place one foot on the footbar **(C)**

PROGRESSION 2

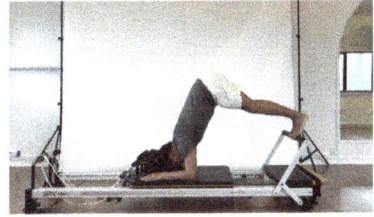

1. Place both feet on the footbar **(C)**

PROGRESSION 3

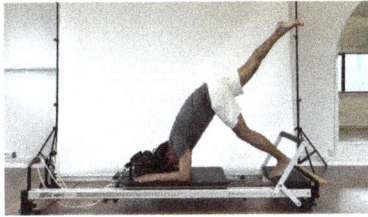

1. Extend one leg up to the ceiling as you lift your hips. The other foot stays on the platform **(C)**

PROGRESSION 4

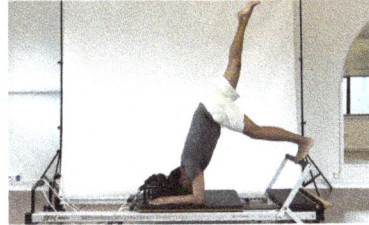

1. Place both feet on the footbar and extend one leg up toward the ceiling as you lift the hips **(C)**

ARMAGEDDON

Strength: Chest, shoulders, abs, quads, glutes, hamstrings

Level: Advanced   **Repetition:** 8-10   **Springs:** Light to medium

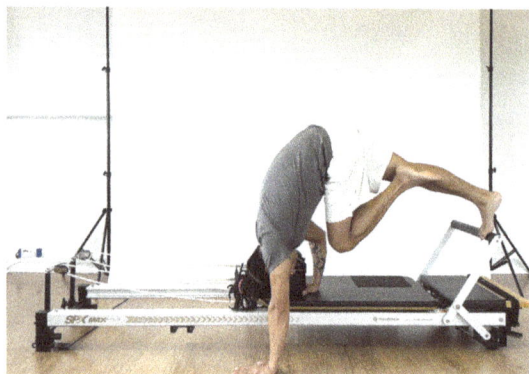

A
START

1. Place one hand on the floor next to the carriage and the other in front of the shoulder rest closest to you.
2. Place the foot closest to the carriage on the footbar and extend the carriage out until the leg is straight.
3. Flex your spine and bring the outer knee forward to the floor arm.

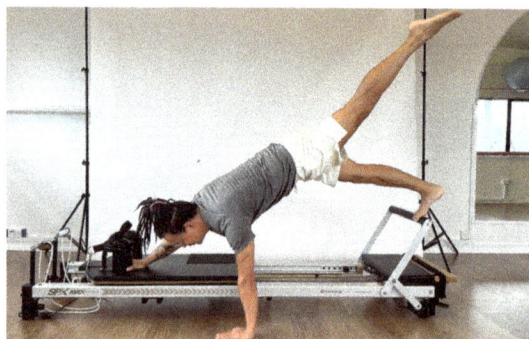

B
EXHALE

1. Push the carriage out, extending your elbow and leg at the same time as you extend your spine.

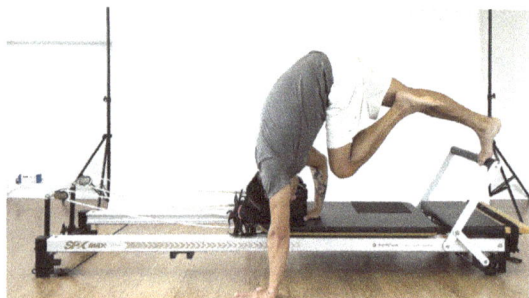

C
INHALE

1. Return to position **A**.
2. Repeat on the other side.

VARIATION

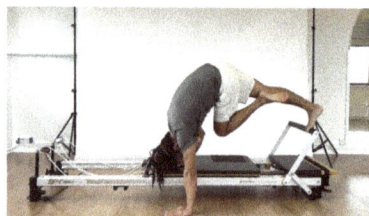

1. Cross the knee over to the carriage elbow **(C)**

KAMIKAZE

Strength: Chest, shoulders, obliques, quads

Level: Advanced   **Repetition:** 8-10   **Springs:** Medium to light

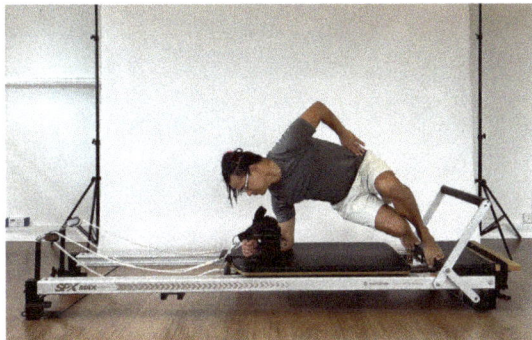

A
START

1. Neutral, four point kneeling position.
2. One elbow is on the carriage at the shoulder rest. Place the other hand on your hip.
3. Place your feet on the inside of the reformer frame or standing platform.
4. Lift both knees off the carriage.

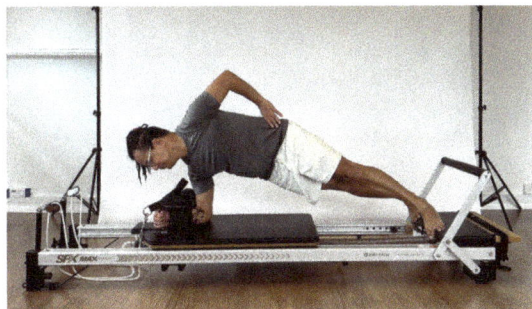

B
EXHALE

1. Extend both your legs, opening the carriage.

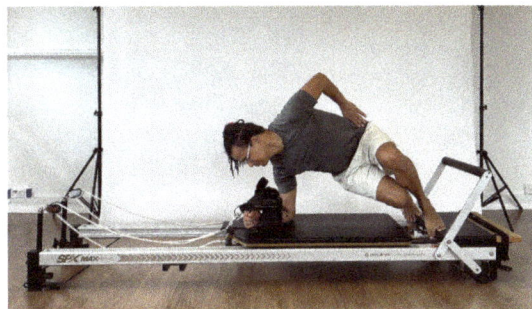

C
INHALE

1. Return to position **A**.
2. Repeat on the other side.

PROGRESSION 1

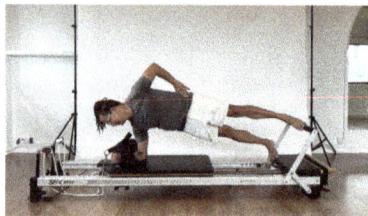

1. Place one foot on the footbar **(B)**

PROGRESSION 2

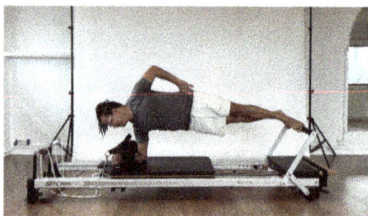

1. Place both feet on the footbar **(B)**

PROGRESSION 3

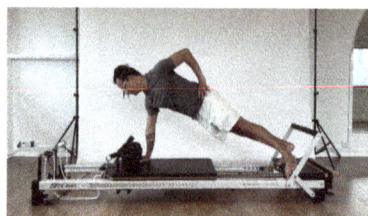

1. Place your hand on the carriage straightening your elbow **(B)**

PROGRESSION 4

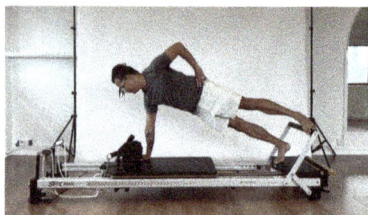

1. Place one foot on the footbar **(B)**

PROGRESSION 5

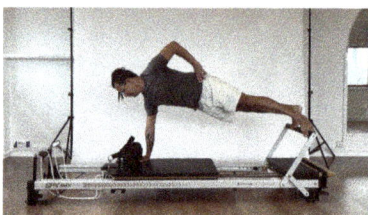

1. Place both feet on the footbar **(B)**

MODIFICATION

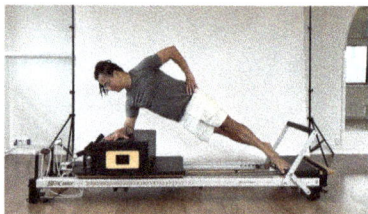

1. Place your elbow on the box **(B)**

PICK AND THROW

Strength: Chest, shoulders, abs, quads, inner thighs

Level: Advanced   **Repetition:** 8-10   **Springs:** Medium

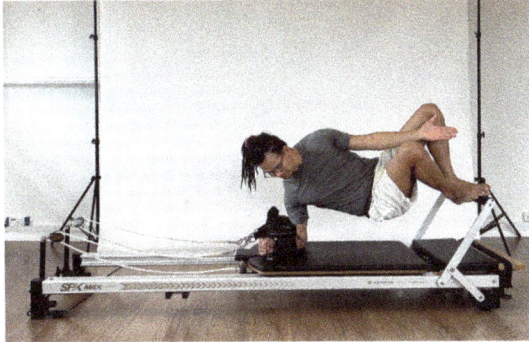

A
START

1. Face sideways placing one forearm on the carriage in front of the shoulder rest.
2. Place your heels on the edge of the footbar with your legs in frog position.
3. Place your hand on your knee.
4. Your hips are suspended above the carriage.

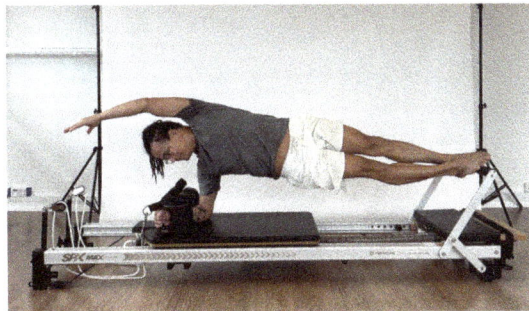

B
EXHALE

1. Extend your legs opening the carriage.
2. Arc your upper hand overhead

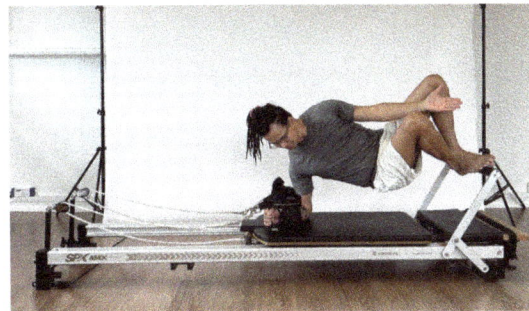

C
INHALE

1. Return to position **A**
2. Repeat on the other side

ARMADILLO I

Strength: Chest, lats, shoulders,arms, abs, quads

Level: Intermediate   **Repetition:** 8-10   **Springs:** Light to medium

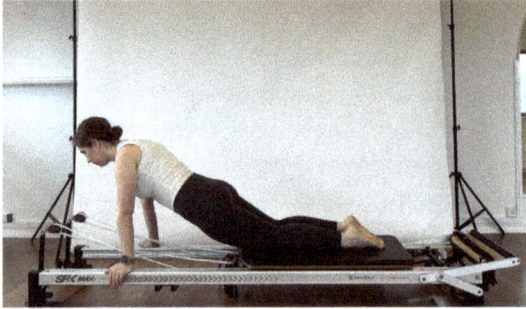

A
START

1. Plank position on your knees. Place your hands on the reformer frame
2. Your knees are placed on the carriage.

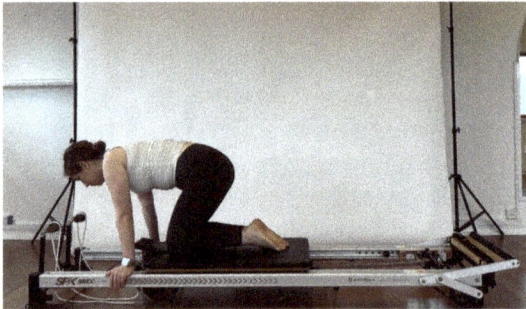

B
EXHALE

1. Pull your knees to your wrists, curving your spine.

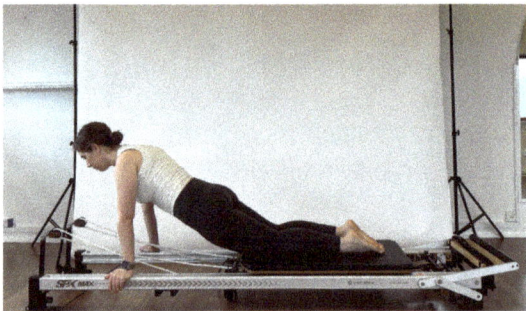

C
INHALE

1. Return to position **A**

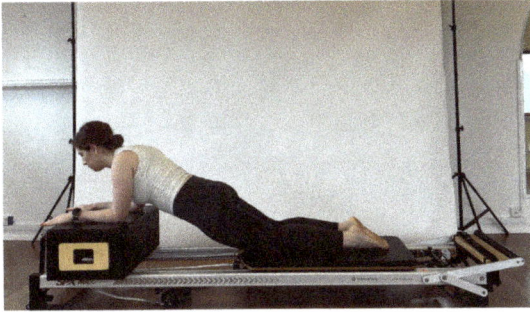

MODIFICATION

1. Place your forearms on top of the box

PROGRESSION 1

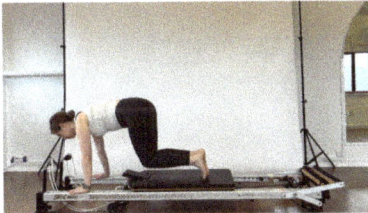

1. Float your knees off the carriage **(B)**

PROGRESSION 2

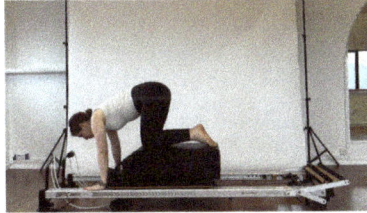

1. Place your knees on top of the box **(B)**

PROGRESSION 3

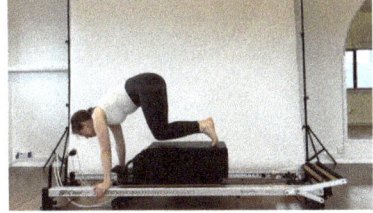

1. Float your knees off the box **(B)**

ARMADILLO II

Strength: Chest, lats, shoulders, arms, abs, quads

Level: Advanced   **Repetition:** 8-10   **Springs:** Light to medium

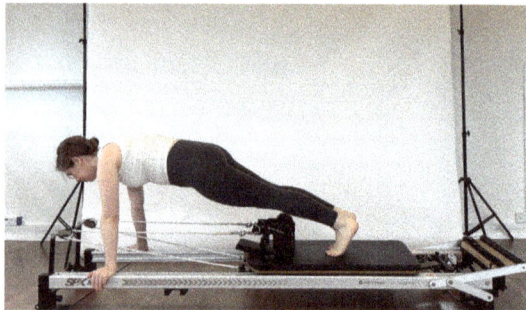

A
START

1. Neutral plank position with your hands on the reformer frame facing the risers.
2. Your feet are on the carriage.

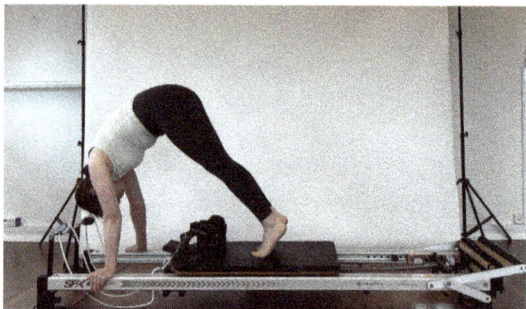

B
EXHALE

1. Pull the carriage towards your hands while lifting your hips to the ceiling and flexing your lower spine.

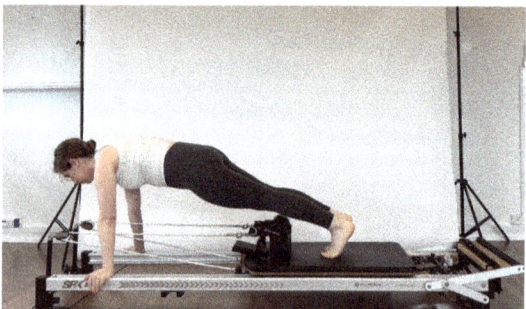

C
INHALE

1. Return to position **A**

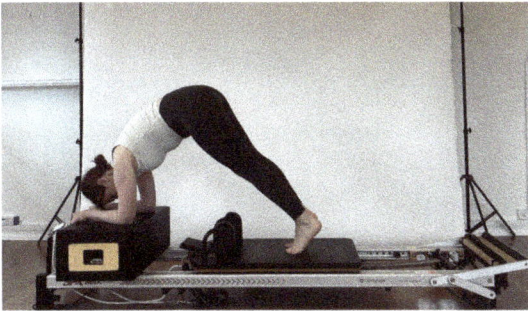

MODIFICATION

1. Place your forearms on top of the box with the box sitting across the frame in front of the risers.

PROGRESSION

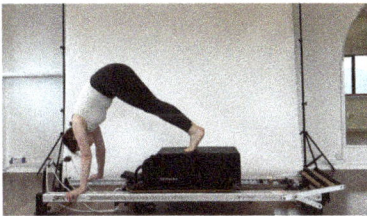

1. Place your feet on top of the box in the long box position. **(B)**

ARMADILLO III

Strength: Chest, lats, shoulders, arms, abs, quads

Level: Advanced   **Repetition:** 8-10   **Springs:** Light to medium

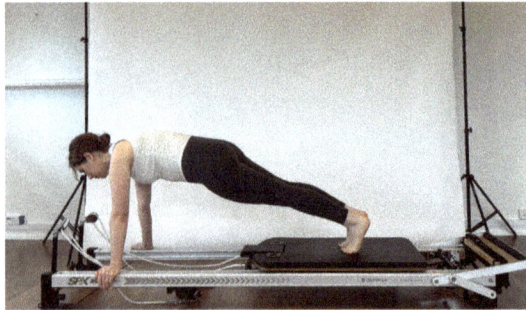

A
START

1. Neutral plank position with your hands on the reformer frame facing the risers.
2. Your feet are on the carriage.

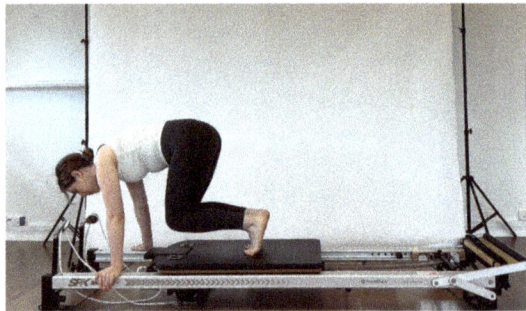

B
EXHALE

1. Pull the carriage towards your hands while bending the knees.
2. Flex your spine.

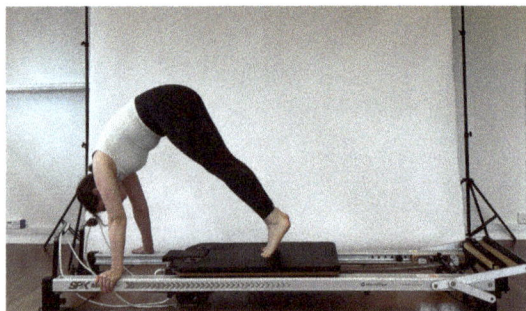

C
INHALE

1. Lift your hips up to the ceiling without moving the carriage.

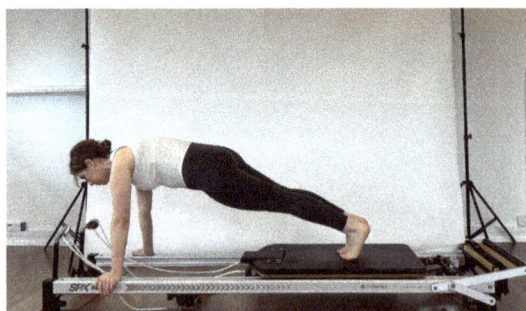

D
EXHALE

1. Return to position **A**

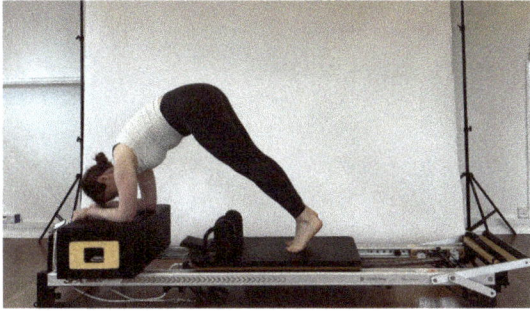

MODIFICATION

1. Place your forearms on top of the box. The box is placed over the frame in the short box position in front of the risers.

PROGRESSION

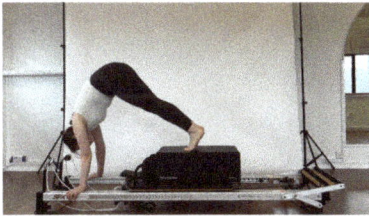

1. Place your feet on top of the box. The box is in the long box position on the carriage **(B)**.

ARMADILLO IV

Strength: Chest, lats, shoulders, arms, abs, quads, glutes, hamstrings

Level: Advanced   **Repetition:** 8-10   **Springs:** Light to medium

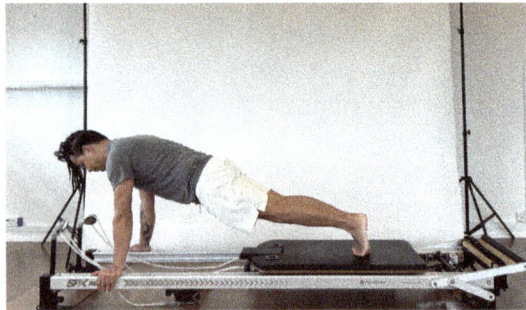

A
START

1. Neutral plank position with your hands on the reformer frame facing the risers.
2. Your feet are on the carriage.

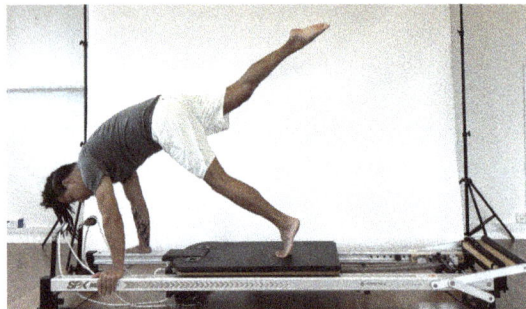

B
EXHALE

1. Pull the carriage towards your hands while lifting one leg up.

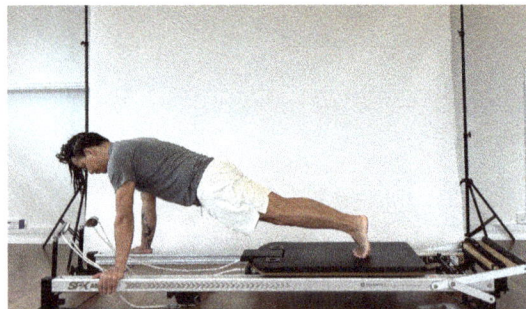

C
INHALE

1. Return to position **A**

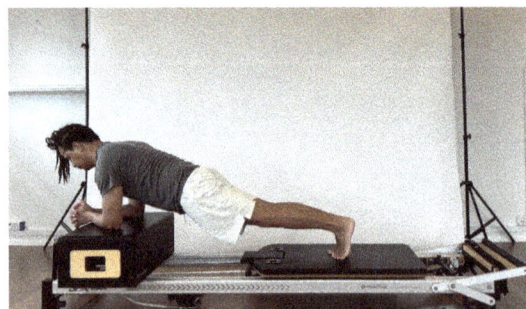

MODIFICATION

1. Place your forearms on top of the box. The box is placed over the frame in the short box position in front of the risers.

THE DRAG I

Strength: Chest, arms, obliques, quads, inner thighs

Level: Intermediate   **Repetition:** 8-10   **Springs:** Light to medium

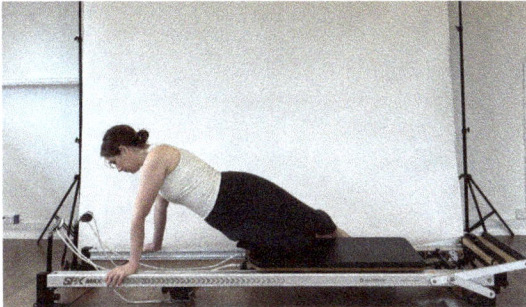

A
START

1. Face the risers and place both hands on the frame
2. Place your thighs on the headrest. Your knees face sideways. Your spine is in a twist.

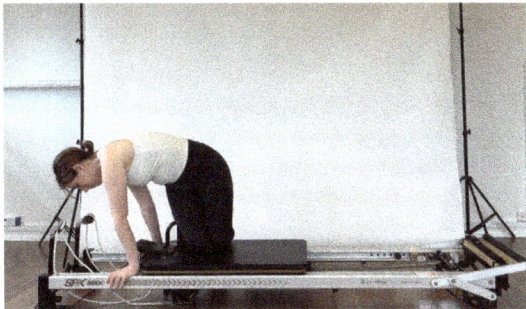

B
EXHALE

1. Pull the carriage towards your hands
2. Lift your hips up at the same time curving your lower spine.

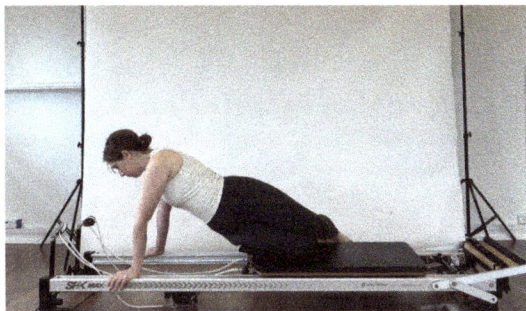

C
INHALE

1. Return to position **A**
2. Repeat on the other side

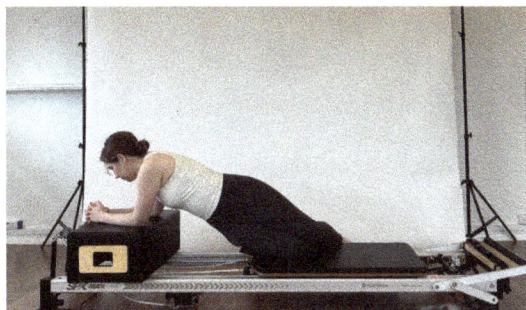

MODIFICATION

1. Elbows on top of the box

THE DRAG II

Strength: Chest, arms, oblique, glutes, quads, inner thighs

Level: Intermediate **Repetition:** 8-10 **Springs:** Light to medium

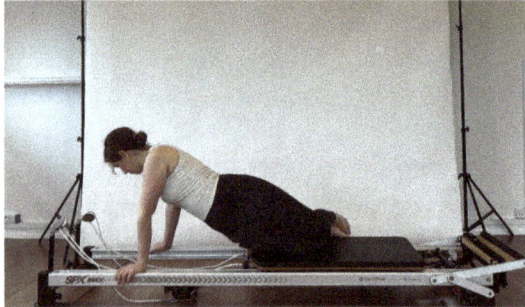

A
START

1. Face the risers and place both hands on the frame
2. Place your thighs on the headrest. Your knees face sideways. Your spine is in a twist.

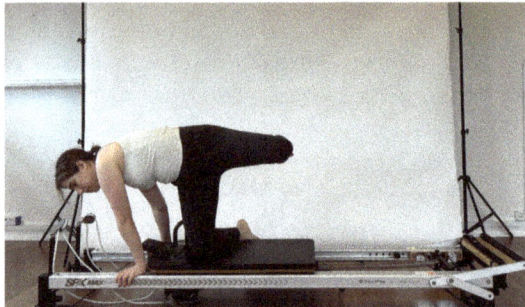

B
EXHALE

1. Pull the carriage towards your hands and lift your hips and outer leg.

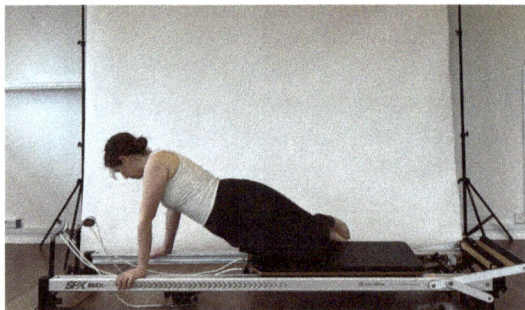

C
INHALE

1. Return to position **A**
2. Repeat on the other side

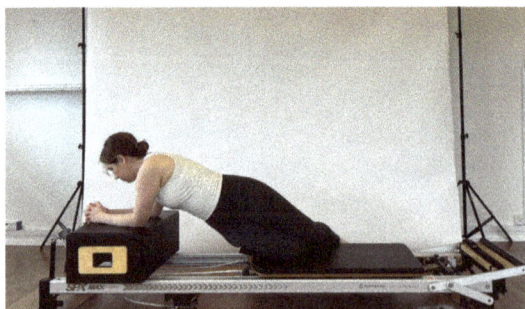

MODIFICATION

1. Elbows on top of the box

THE DRAG III

Strength: Chest, arms, oblique, glutes, quads, inner thighs

Level: Intermediate   **Repetition:** 8-10   **Springs:** Light to medium

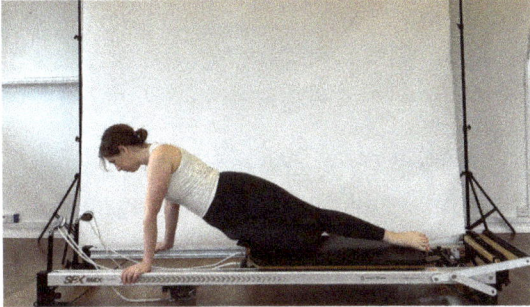

A
START

1. Face the risers and place both hands on the frame
2. Place your thighs on the headrest. Your knees face sideways. Your spine is in a twist.
3. Extend the upper leg straight and in line with your hip

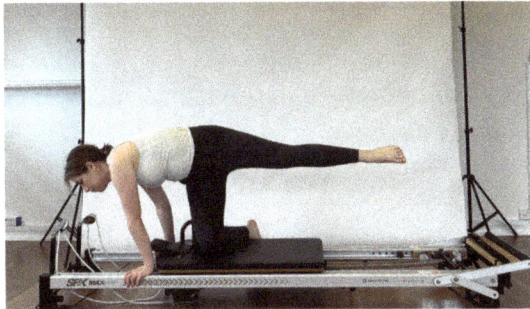

B
EXHALE

1. Pull the carriage towards your hands while lifting your hips and outer leg.

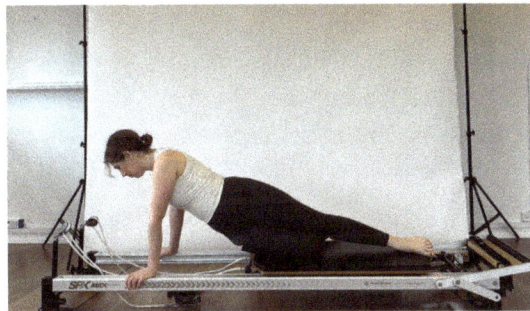

C
INHALE

1. Return to position **A**
2. Repeat on the other side

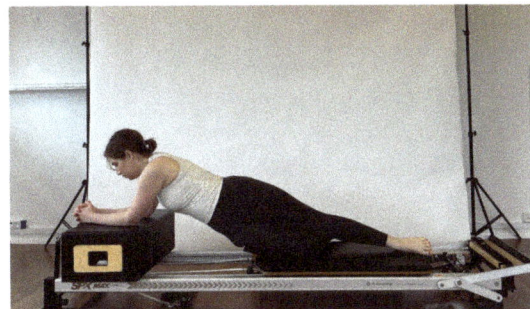

MODIFICATION

1. Elbows on top of the box

EXCALIBUR I

Strength: Chest, arms, obliques, quads, inner thigh

Level: Advanced   **Repetition:** 8-10   **Springs:** Light to medium

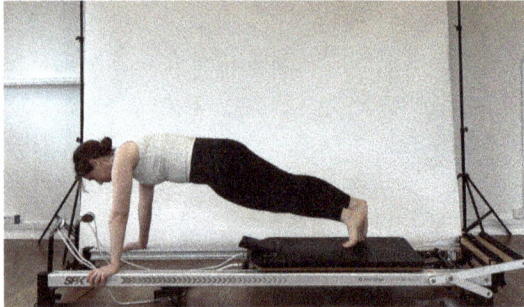

A
START

1. Face the risers and place both hands on the frame
2. Extend your legs and cross one leg over the other in an oblique plank position

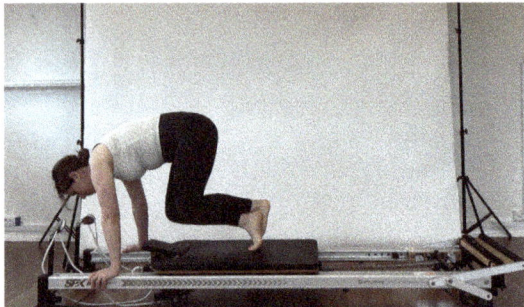

B
EXHALE

1. Pull the carriage in by bending your knees towards your arms.
2. Keep your knees off the carriage

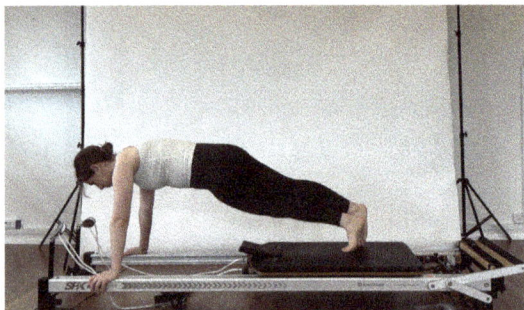

C
INHALE

1. Return to position **A**
2. Repeat on the other side

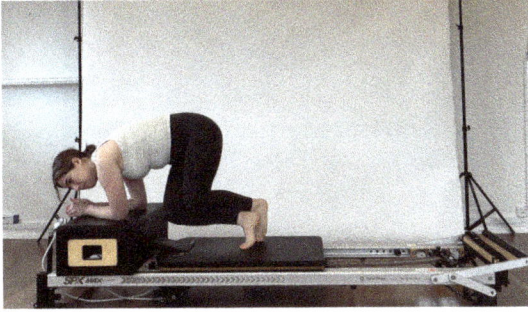

MODIFICATION

1. Elbows on top of the box

VARIATION

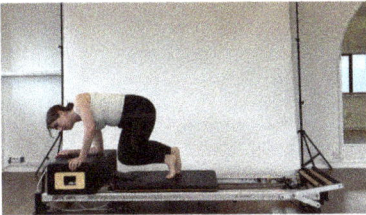

1. Elbow and hands on top of the box **(B)**

EXCALIBUR II

Strength: Chest, arms, obliques, quads, inner thighs

Level: Advanced   **Repetition:** 8-10   **Springs:** Light to medium

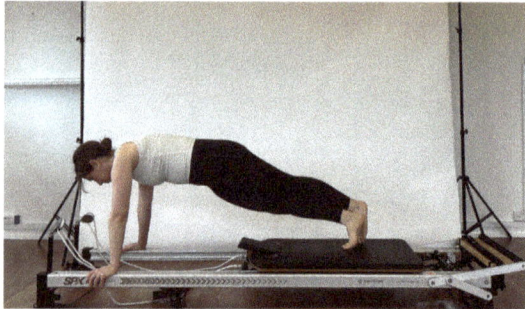

A
START

1. Face the risers and place both hands on the frame
2. Extend your legs and cross one leg over the other in an oblique plank position

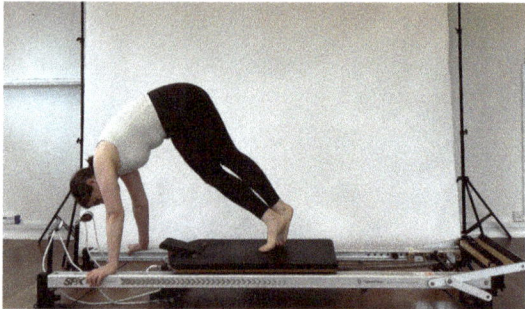

B
EXHALE

1. Pull the carriage towards your arms while lifting both hips to the ceiling.

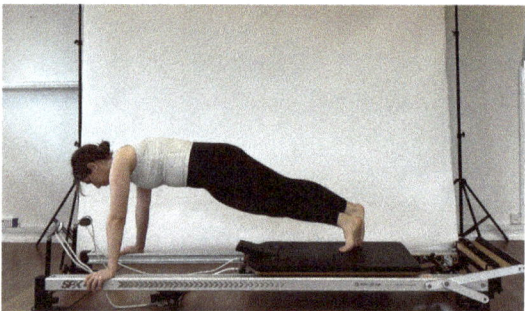

C
INHALE

1. Return to position **A**
2. Repeat on the other side

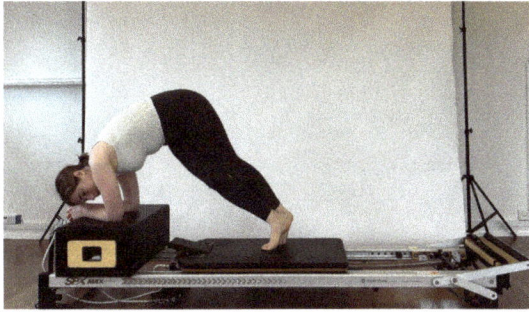

MODIFICATION

1. Elbows on top of the box

VARIATION

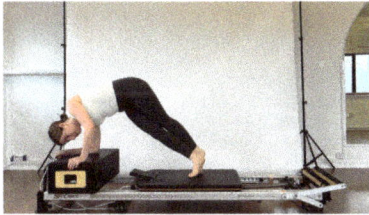

1. Elbow and hands on top of the box **(B)**

EXCALIBUR III

Strength: Chest, arms, oblique, quads, inner thigh

Level: Advance   **Repetition:** 8-10   **Springs:** light to medium

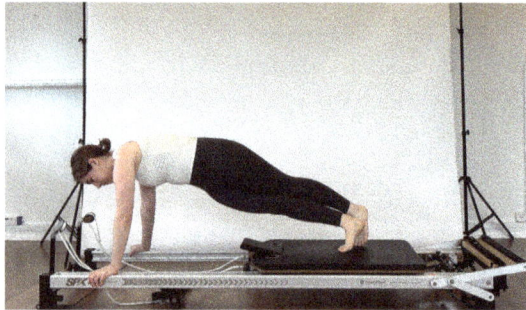

A
START

1. Face the risers and place both hands on the frame.
2. Extend your legs and cross one leg over the other in an oblique plank position.

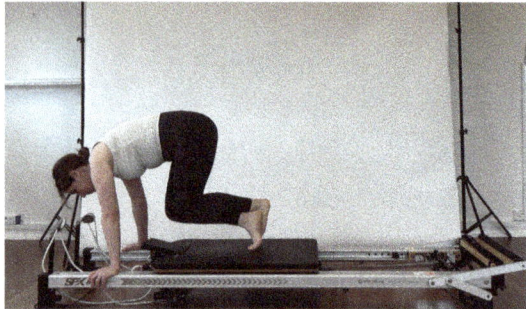

B
EXHALE

1. Pull the carriage toward your arms and bend both knees. Keep your knees off the carriage.

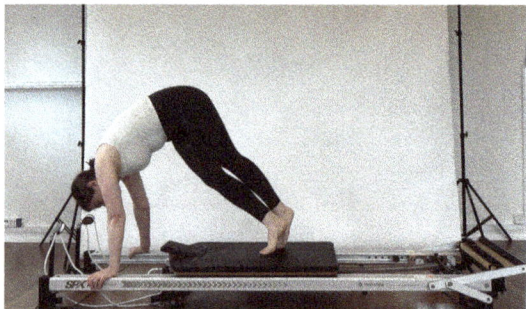

C
INHALE

1. Lift your hips, straightening your legs without moving the carriage.
2. Pull the carriage towards your arms.

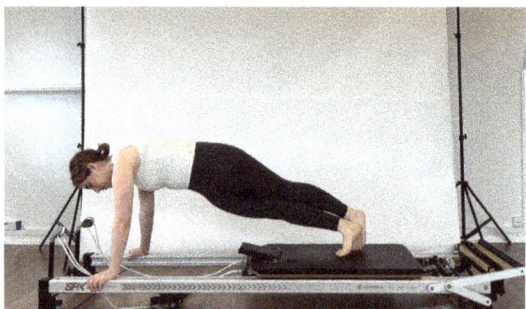

D
EXHALE

1. Return to position **A**
2. Repeat on the other side

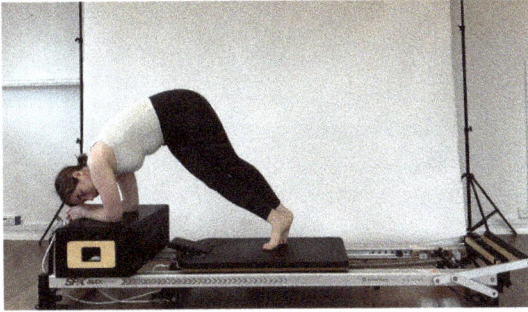

MODIFICATION

1. Elbows on top of the box

VARIATION

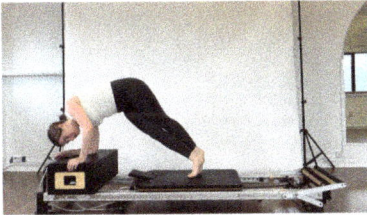

1. Elbow and hands on top of the box **(C)**

SLEEPOVER I

Strength: Shoulder, oblique, inner thigh

Level: Advance   **Repetition:** 8-10   **Springs:** light to medium

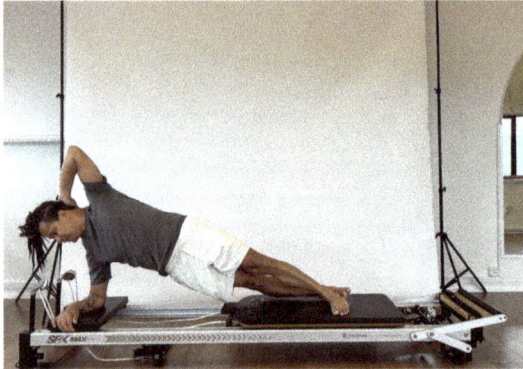

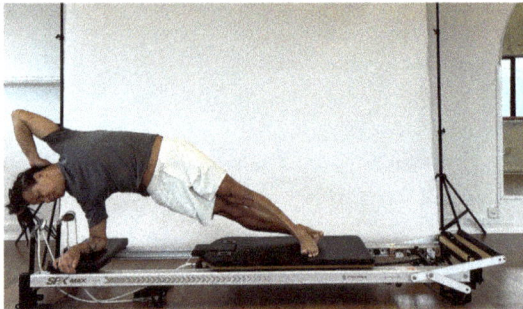

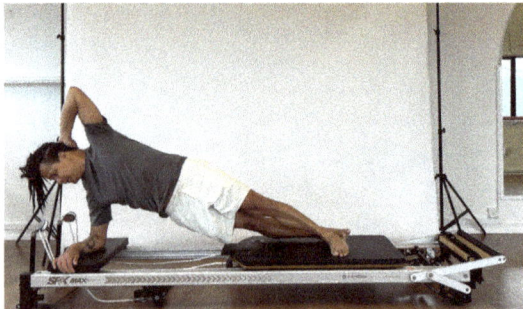

A
START

1. Place a platform extender at the riser end of your reformer.
2. Place your forearm on the extender.
3. Your body is in a side plank position with your legs extended and your lower leg in front of the upper leg.
4. Place your upper hand at the back of your head.

B
EXHALE

1. Lift your hips up to the ceiling as you pull the carriage towards the platform extender

C
INHALE

1. Return to position **A**
2. Repeat on the other side

SLEEPOVER II

Strength: Shoulders, obliques, inner thighs

Level: Advanced   **Repetition:** 8-10   **Springs:** Light to medium

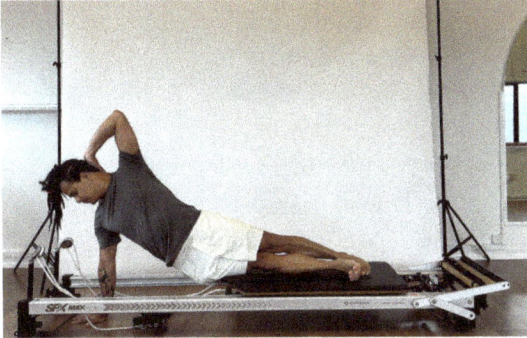

A
START

1. Lie down on your side. Place your lower hand on the floor into the well of the reformer. Extend your arm.
2. Place your lower leg in front of the upper leg. Both legs are fully extended.
3. Place the upper hand behind your head.
4. Rest your hips on top of the headrest.

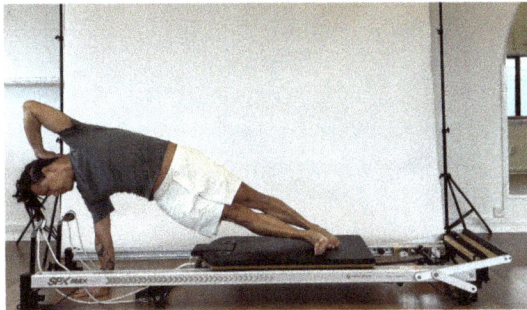

B
EXHALE

1. Lift your hips up to the ceiling while pulling the carriage towards the supporting arm.

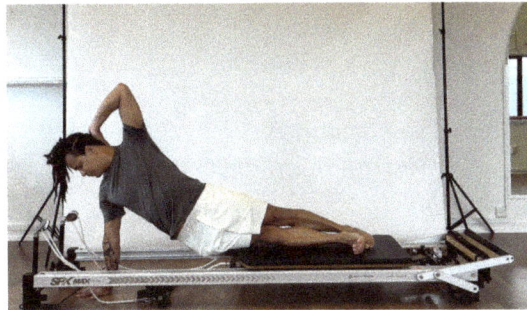

C
INHALE

1. Return to position **A**
2. Repeat on the other side

BROKEN ARROW I

Strength: Shoulders, obliques, quads, inner thighs

Level: Advanced   **Repetition:** 8-10   **Springs:** Light to medium

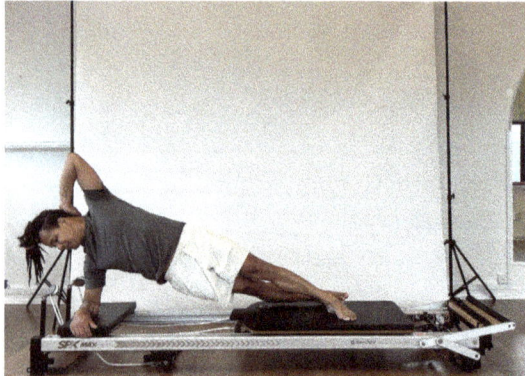

A
START

1. Place a platform extender at the riser end of your reformer.
2. Place your forearm on the extender.
3. Your body is in a side plank position with your legs extended and hips lifted. Your lower leg is in front of the upper leg.
4. Place your upper hand at the back of your head.

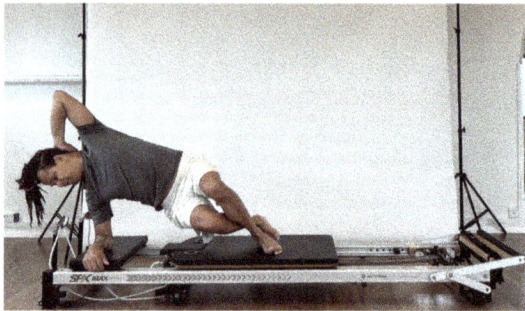

B
EXHALE

1. Pull the carriage towards your supporting arm as you bend your knees.

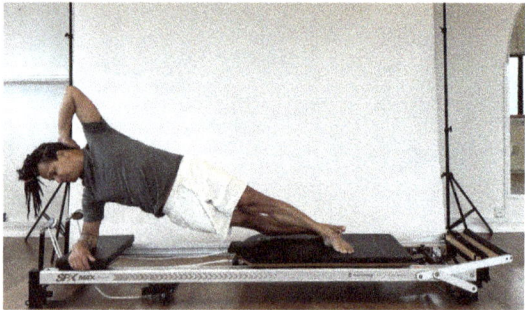

C
INHALE

1. Return to position **A**
2. Repeat on the other side

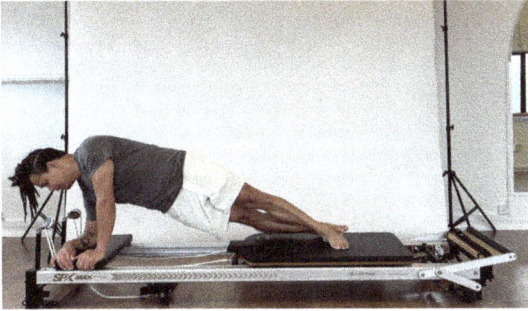

MODIFICATION

1. Hands and elbow on the platform

PROGRESSION

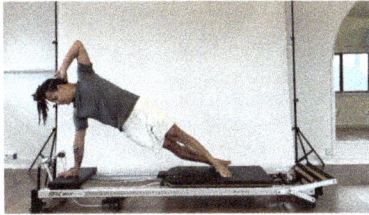

1. Extend the supporting arm. Place the weight on your hand **(A)**

MODIFICATION

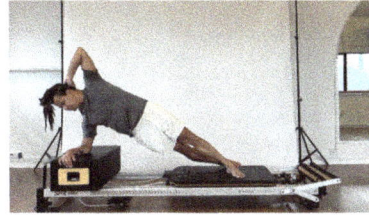

1. Forearm on top of the box **(A)**

BROKEN ARROW II

Strength: Shoulders, obliques, quads, inner thighs

Level: Advanced **Repetition:** 8-10 **Springs:** Light to medium

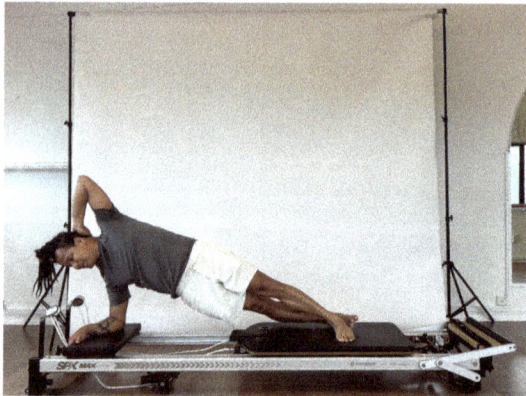

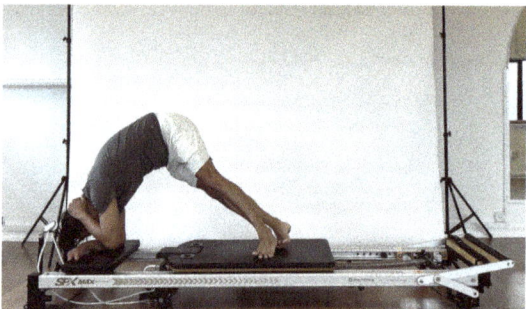

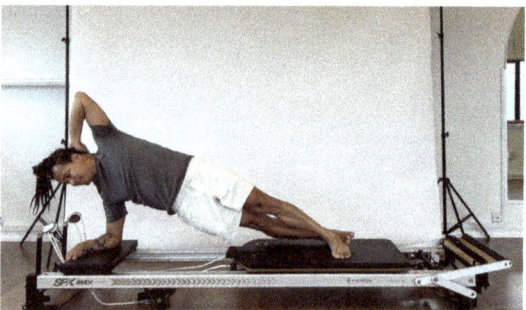

A
START

1. Place a platform extender at the riser end of your reformer.
2. Place your forearm on the extender.
3. Your body is in a side plank position with your legs extended and your lower leg in front of the upper leg. Your hips are elevated.
4. Place your upper hand at the back of your head.

B
EXHALE

1. Lift your hips up to the ceiling keeping your legs straight.
2. Rotate your spine so your upper elbow reaches for your lower hand.

C
INHALE

1. Return to position **A**
2. Repeat on the other side.

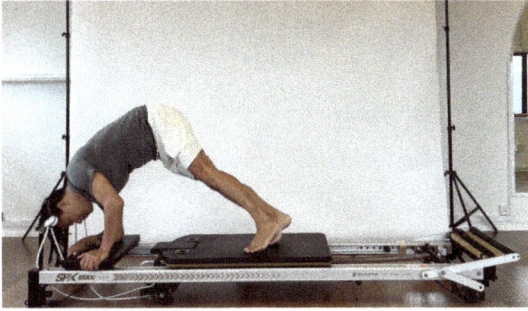

MODIFICATION

1. Place your upper hand on the platform

PROGRESSION

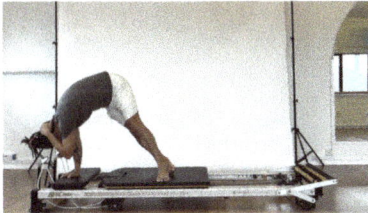

1. Extend arm on the platform **(B)**

MODIFICATION

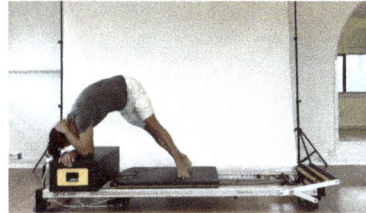

1. Place one elbow on top of the box **(B)**

THE FROG PRINCESS I

Strength: Chest, lats, shoulders, abs, quads

Level: Advanced   **Repetition:** 8-10   **Springs:** Light to medium

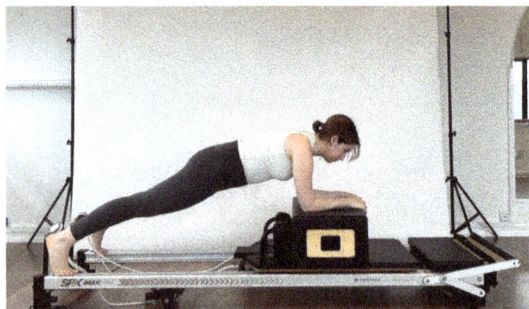

A
START

1. Plank position facing the footbar.
2. Place your elbows on top of the reformer box with both legs extended. Your feet are placed on the frame.

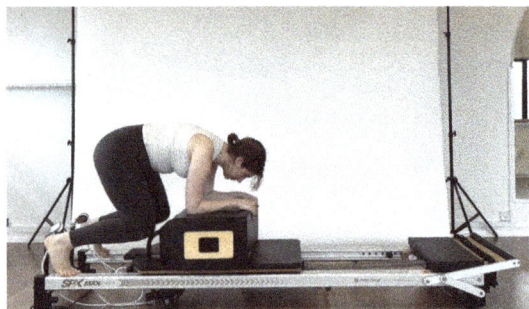

B
EXHALE

1. Bend your knees and pull the carriage toward you.
2. Transfer your weight to your legs and 'sit' on your heels.
3. At the same time draw your belly in and shoulders down, curving your spine

C
INHALE

1. Return to position **A**

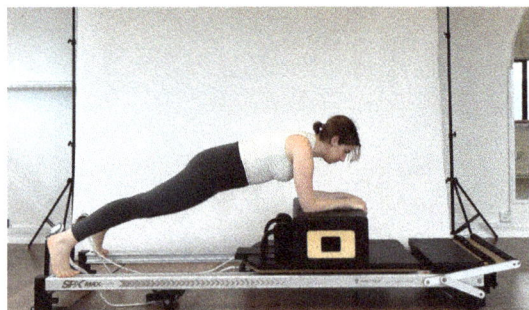

PROGRESSION 1

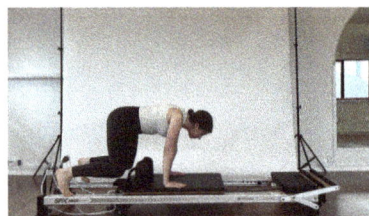

1. Both arms are straight with your hands in front of the shoulder rests **(B)**

PROGRESSION 2

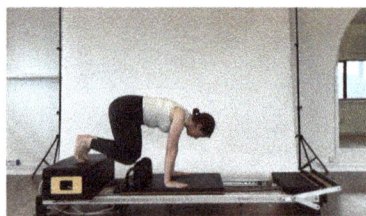

1. Place your feet on top of the box **(B)**

THE FROG PRINCESS II

Strength: Chest, lats, shoulders, abs, quads

Level: Advanced **Repetition:** 8-10 **Springs:** Light to medium

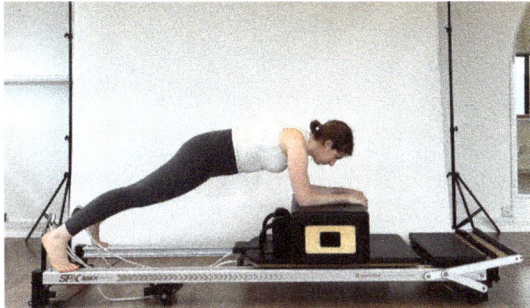

A
START

1. Plank position facing the footbar.
2. Place your elbows on top of the reformer box with both legs extended. Your feet are placed on the frame.

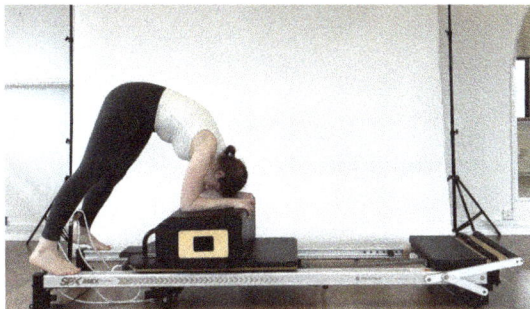

B
EXHALE

1. Lift your hips toward the ceiling curving your spine. Keep your legs straight.

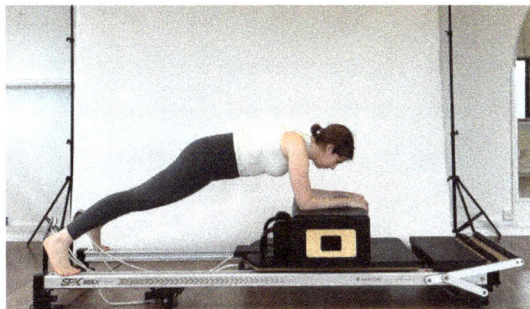

C
INHALE

1. Return to position **A**

PROGRESSION 1

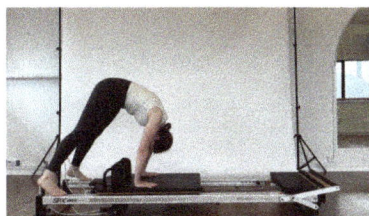

1. Both arms are straight with your hands in front of the shoulder rests **(B)**

PROGRESSION 2

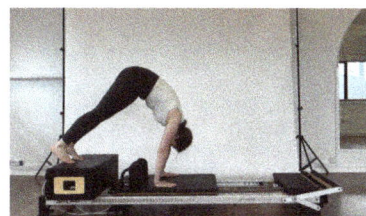

1. Place your feet on top of the box **(B)**

THE FROG PRINCESS III

Strength: Chest, lats, shoulders, abs, quads

Level: Advanced   **Repetition:** 8-10   **Springs:** Light to medium

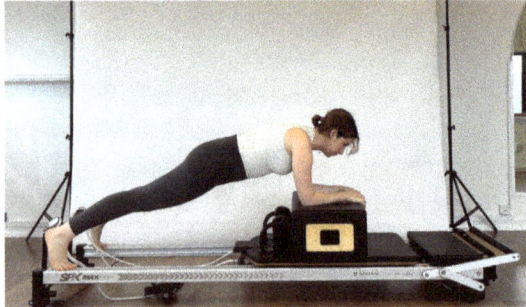

A
START

1. Plank position facing the footbar.
2. Place your elbows on top of the reformer box with both legs extended. Your feet are placed on the frame.

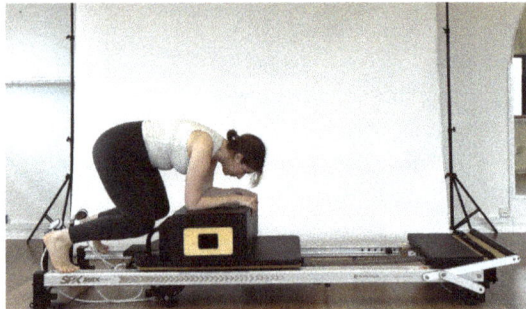

B

EXHALE

1. Bend your knees pulling your body toward your legs.

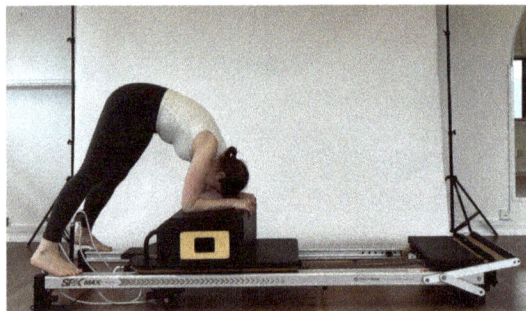

C
INHALE

1. Lift your hips to the ceiling without moving the carriage. Press your heels down.

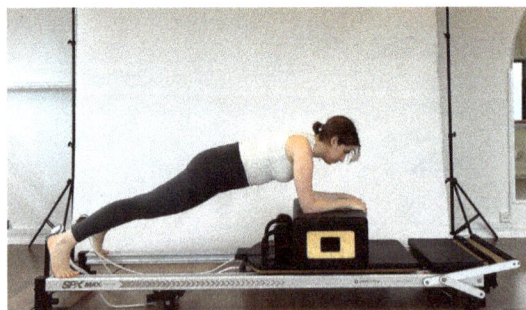

D
EXHALE

1. Return to position **A**

PROGRESSION 1

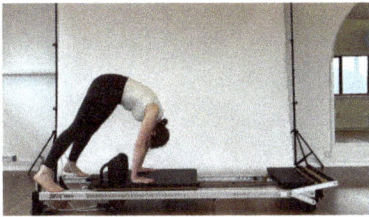

1. Both arms are straight with your hands in front of the shoulder rests **(B)**

PROGRESSION 2

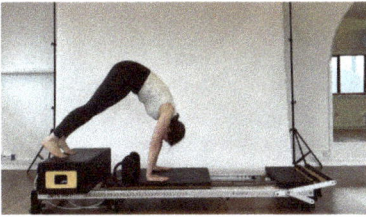

1. Place your feet on top of the box **(B)**

UNTOLD
PART III

DEAD CABLE I

Strength: Back, arms, shoulders, abs, glutes, quads, hamstrings, calves

Level: Intermediate   **Repetition:** 8-10   **Springs:** medium to heavy

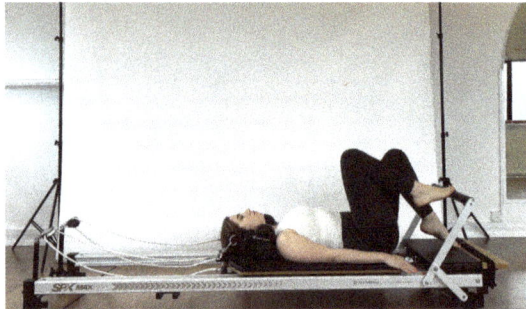

A

START

1. Lie on your back on the carriage.
2. Place the ball of one foot on the footbar.
3. Place the other foot on the standing platform on the ball of the foot. The heel is raised.

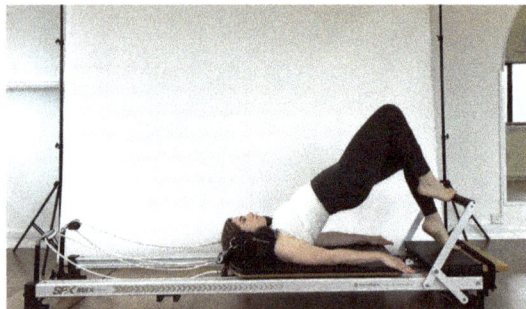

B

EXHALE

1. Articulate the spine up to a bridge position.

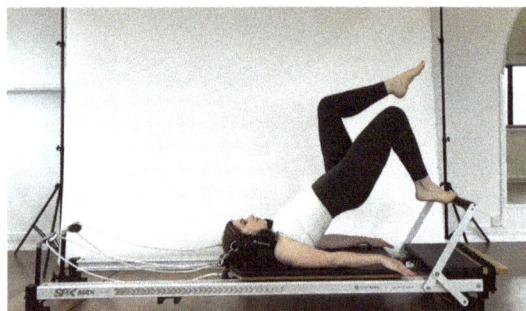

C

INHALE

1. Lift the lower leg to table top position.

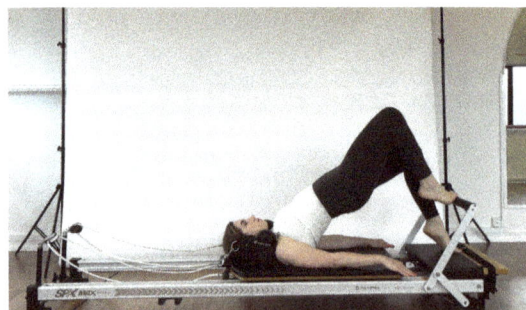

D

EXHALE

1. Reverse the leg movement.

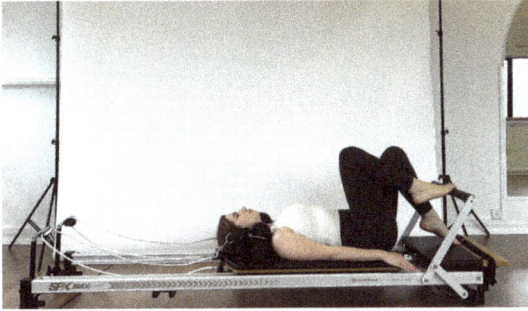

E
INHALE

1. Return to position **A**
2. Repeat on the other side

PROGRESSION

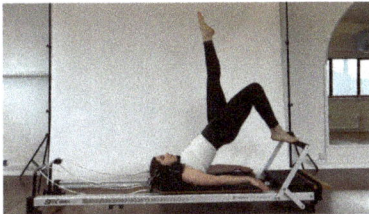

1. Extend the gesture leg, toes point to the ceiling **(C)**

DEAD CABLE II

Strength: Arms, shoulders, abs, glutes, quads, hamstrings

Level: Intermediate   **Repetition:** 8-10   **Springs:** Medium

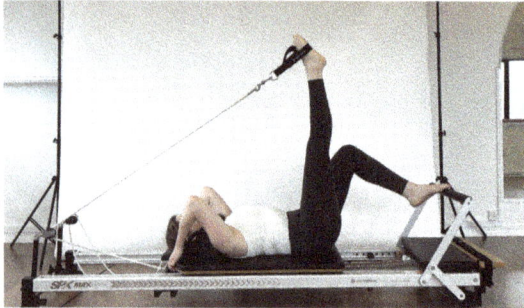

A
START

1. Lie on your back on the carriage.
2. Hold onto the back of the carriage with your hands
3. Place one foot in the strap, extending your leg.
4. Place the heel of the other foot on the footbar.

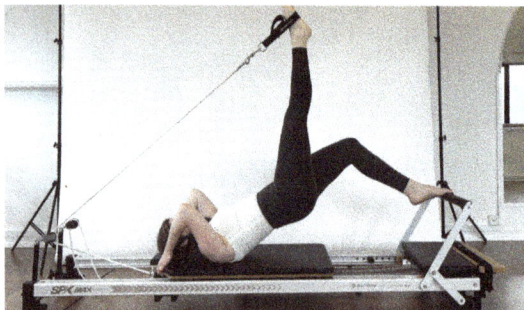

B
EXHALE

1. Articulate your spine up to the bridge position. Keep your extended leg reaching up toward the ceiling.
2. Shoulder draw down toward the footbar slightly.

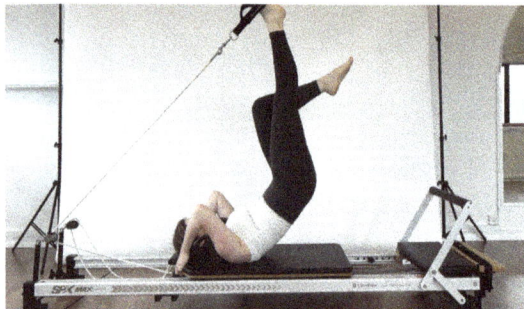

C
INHALE

1. Lift the lower leg to table top as you draw your shoulders down more and press your hands into the carriage frame to keep you steady.

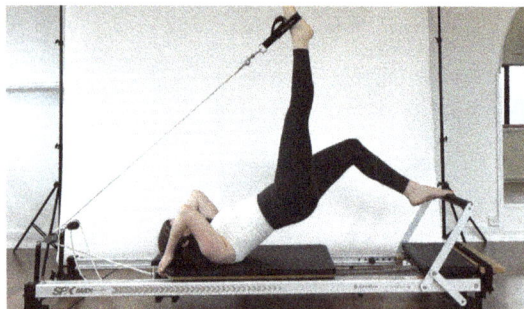

D
EXHALE

1. Place your foot back on the footbar.

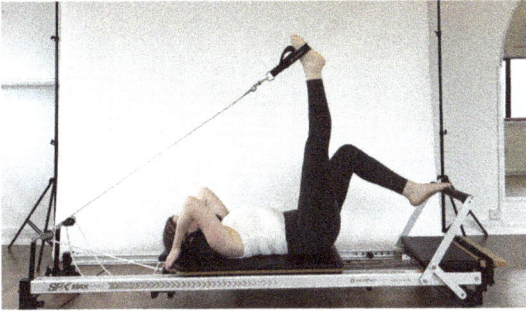

E
INHALE

1. Articulate your spine down to position **A**
2. Repeat on the other side

PROGRESSION 1

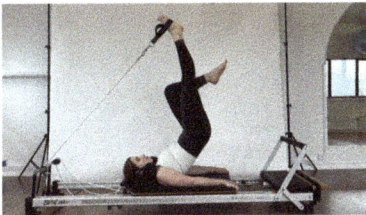

1. Place both arms on carriage next to your body **(C)**

PROGRESSION 2

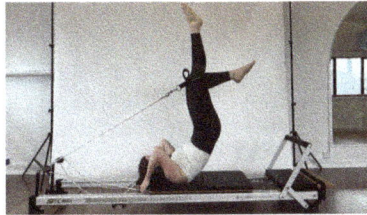

1. Place the footbar leg into the strap behind your knee. The other leg is extended up to the ceiling without a strap **(C)**

PROGRESSION 3

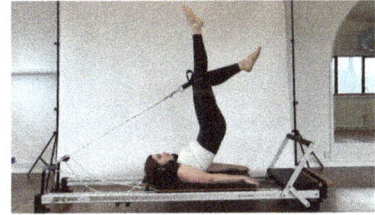

1. Place your arms beside you on the carriage and your knee in the strap **(C)**

THE HANGING BRIDGE I

Strength: arms, shoulders, triceps, abs, bum, quads, hamstring

Level: Intermediate **Repetition:** 8-10 **Springs:** medium

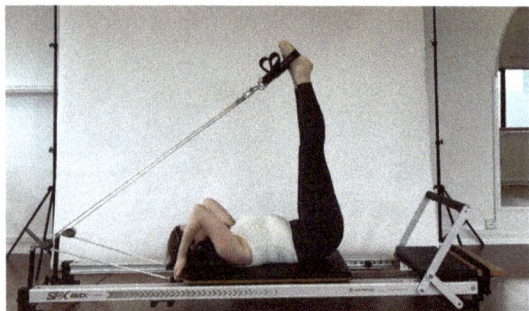

A

STAR

1. Lie on your back with both hands holding the back of the carriage.
2. Your legs can either be together or crossed as they extend up to the ceiling.

Intermediate: Both straps
Advanced: Single strap

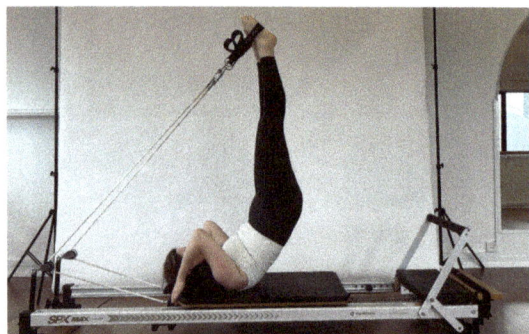

B

EXHALE

1. Articulate your spine to lift your hips up until you reach your shoulder blades.
2. Your legs stay reaching directly up to the ceiling. Draw your shoulders away from the shoulder rests as you press your hands into the carriage.

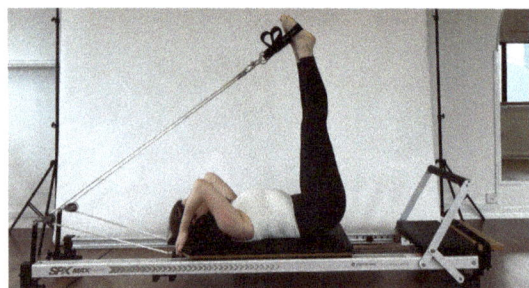

C

INHALE

1. Articulate your spine down to position **A**

PROGRESSION 1

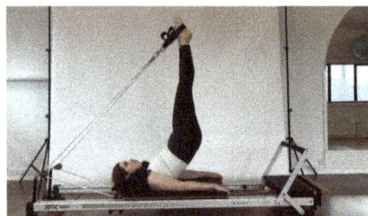

1. Place your arms next to you on the carriage and both feet in the straps **(B)**

PROGRESSION 2

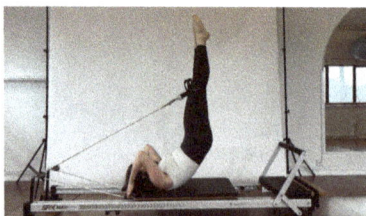

1. Your hands hold on at the back of the carriage. Place your knees in the straps **(B)**

PROGRESSION 3

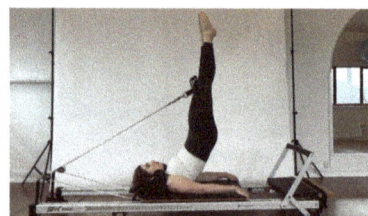

1. Place both arms on the carriage next to your body and knees in the straps **(B)**

THE HANGING BRIDGE II

Strength: Arms, shoulders, triceps, abs, glutes, quads, hamstrings

Level: Intermediate   **Repetition:** 8-10   **Springs:** Medium

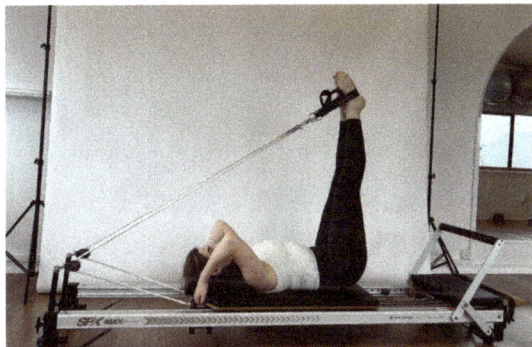

A
START

1. Lie on your back with both hands holding the back of the carriage.
2. Extend both legs up toward the ceiling. You can either keep your legs together or cross one over the other.

Intermediate: Both straps
Advanced: Single strap

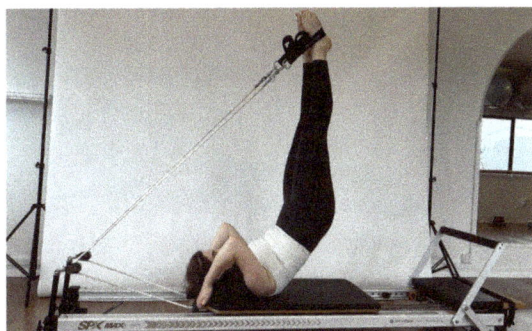

B
EXHALE

1. Articulate up through your spine as you lift your hips to the shoulder blades
2. Draw your shoulders away from the shoulder rests as you press your hands into the carriage.

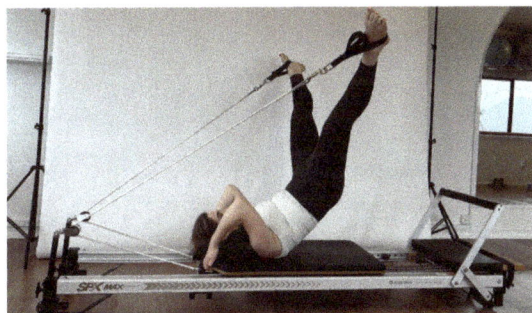

C
INHALE

1. Open your legs sideways.

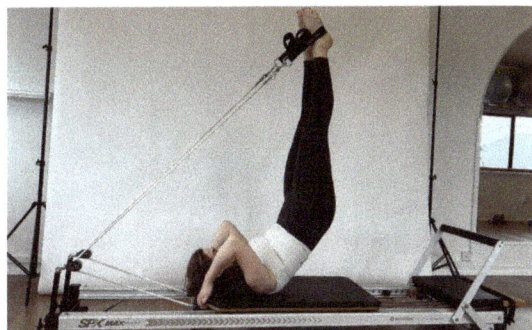

D
EXHALE

1. Close your legs.

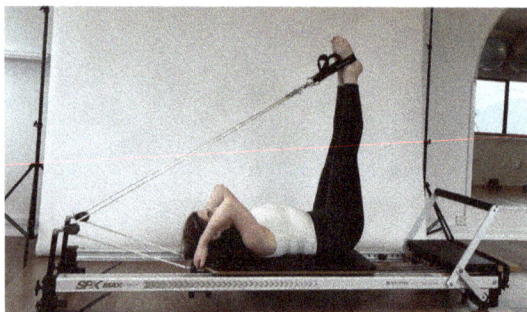

E

INHALE

1. Return to position **A**

PROGRESSION 1

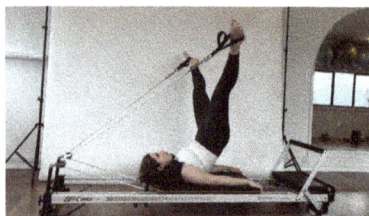

1. Place both arms next to you on the carriage and feet in the straps **(C)**

PROGRESSION 2

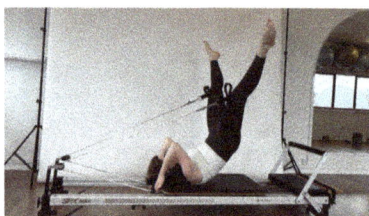

1. Hold onto the back of the carriage and place straps on knees **(C)**

PROGRESSION 3

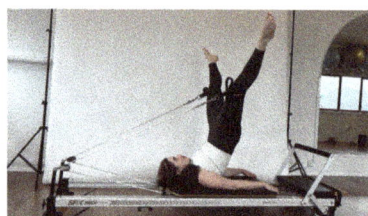

1. Place both arms next to you on the carriage and place strap around knee **(C)**

HYDRAULIC JACK I

Strength: arms, shoulders, triceps, abs, glutes, quads, hamstrings

Level: Advanced   **Repetition:** 8-10   **Springs:** Medium

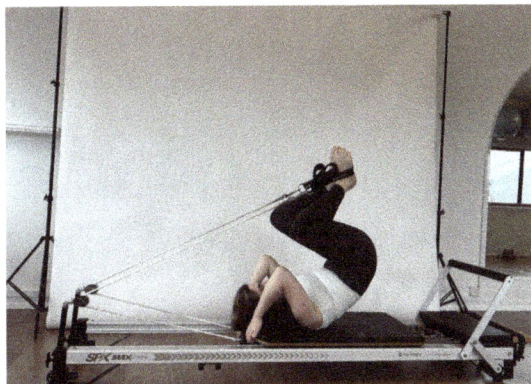

A
START

1. Hold onto the back of the carriage with your hands.
2. Roll over flexing your spine until you reach your shoulders.
3. Your legs are bent in frog position with your knees above your elbows

Intermediate: Both straps
Advanced: Single strap

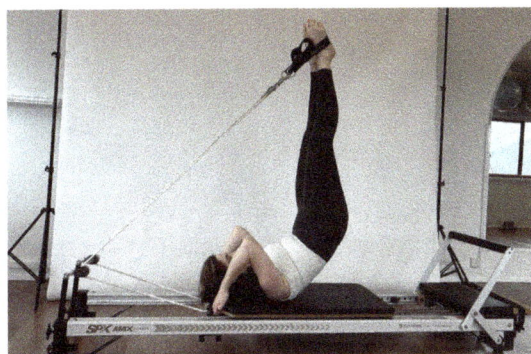

B
EXHALE

1. Extend both legs up to the ceiling.

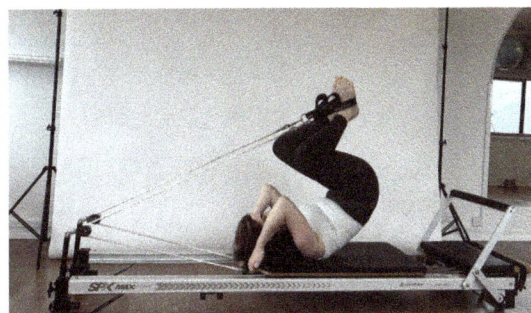

C
INHALE

1. Return to position **A**

PROGRESSION 1

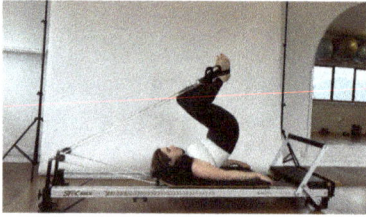

1. Place both arms on the carriage next to your body. Place your feet in the straps **(A)**

PROGRESSION 2

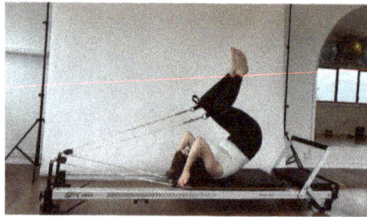

1. Hold onto the back of the carriage with your hands and place the straps around your knees **(A)**

PROGRESSION 3

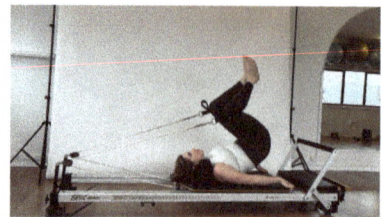

1. Place both arms next to your body on the carriage and the straps around the knees **(A)**

HYDRAULIC JACK II

Strength: Arms, shoulders, triceps, abs, glutes, quads, hamstrings

Level: Advanced   **Repetition:** 8-10   **Springs:** Medium

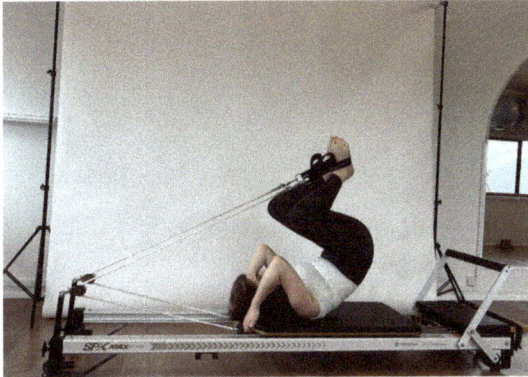

A
START

1. Hold onto the back of the carriage with your hands.
2. Roll over flexing your spine until you reach your shoulders.
3. Your legs are bent in frog position with your knees above your elbows.

Intermediate: Both straps
Advanced: Single strap

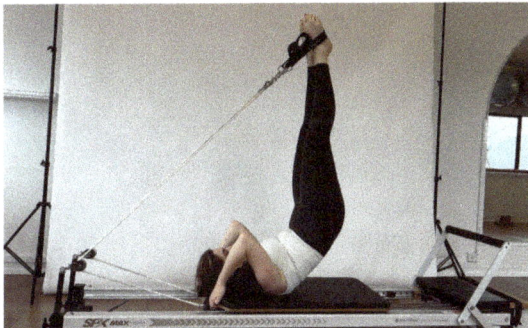

B
EXHALE

1. Extend both legs up to the ceiling.

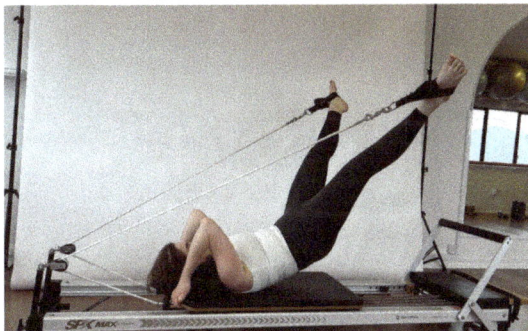

C
INHALE

1. Open your legs sideways.

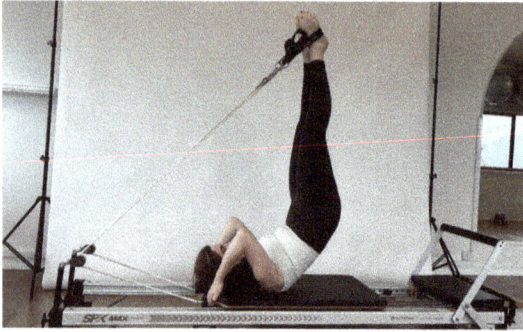

D
EXHALE

1. Close your legs.

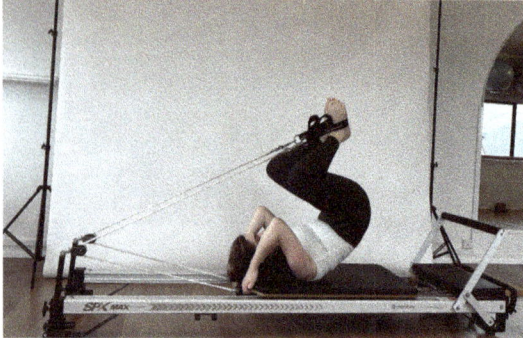

E
INHALE

1. Return to position **A**

PROGRESSION 1

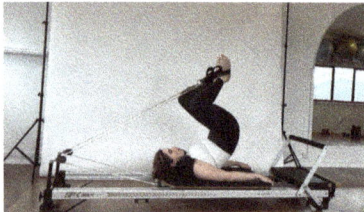

1. Place your arms on the carriage next to your body and feet in the straps **(A)**

PROGRESSION 2

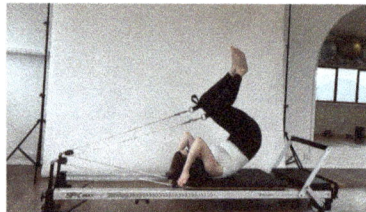

1. Hold onto the back of the carriage with both hands and knees in the straps **(A)**

PROGRESSION 3

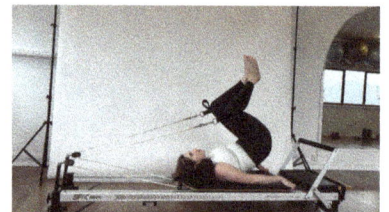

1. Place your arms on the carriage next to your body and knees in the straps **(A)**

HYDRAULIC JACK III

Strength: Arms, shoulders, abs, glutes, quads, hamstrings

Level: Advanced   **Repetition:** 8-10   **Springs:** Medium

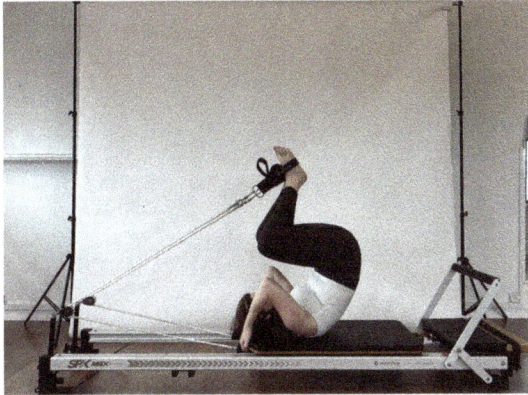

A
START

1. Hold onto the back of the carriage with both hands. Your elbows point up toward the ceiling.
2. Articulate your spine to bring your hips over your shoulders.
3. Bend your legs into the frog position with your knees over your elbows.

Intermediate: Both straps
Advance: Single strap

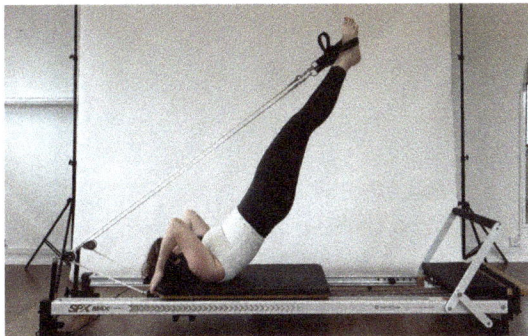

B
EXHALE

1. Extend both legs out to a 45 degree angle. Your spine remains elevated off the carriage.

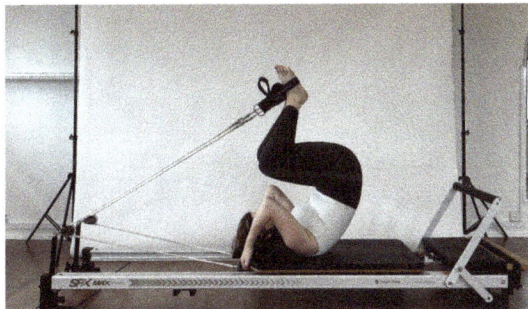

C
INHALE

1. Return to position **A**.

PROGRESSION 1

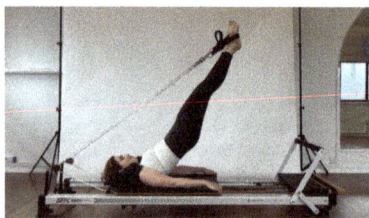

1. Place both arms on the carriage next to your body **(B)**

PROGRESSION 2

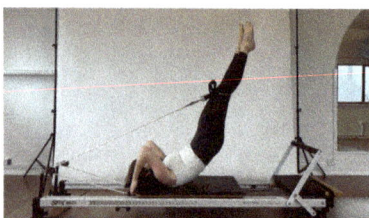

1. Both hands hold onto the back of the carriage and both knees in the straps **(B)**

PROGRESSION 3

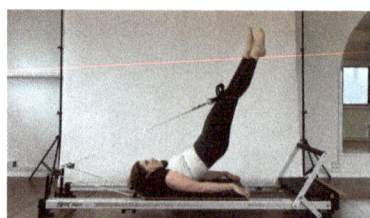

1. Place both arms on the carriage next to your body and both knees in the straps **(B)**

HYDRAULIC JACK IV

Strength: Arms, shoulders, abs, glutes, quads, hamstrings

Level: Advanced   **Repetition:** 8-10   **Springs:** Medium

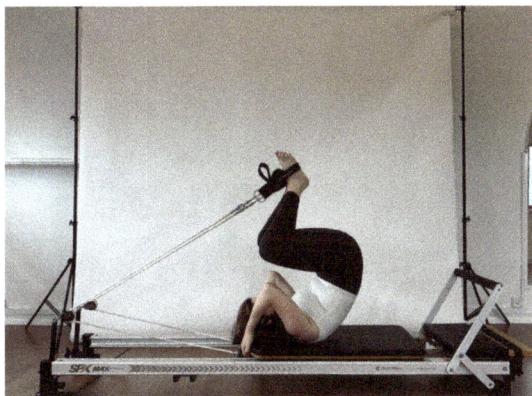

A
START

1. Hold onto the back of the carriage with both hands. Your elbows point up toward the ceiling.
2. Articulate your spine to bring your hips over your shoulders.
3. Bend your legs into the frog position with your knees over your elbows.

Intermediate: Both straps
Advance: Single strap

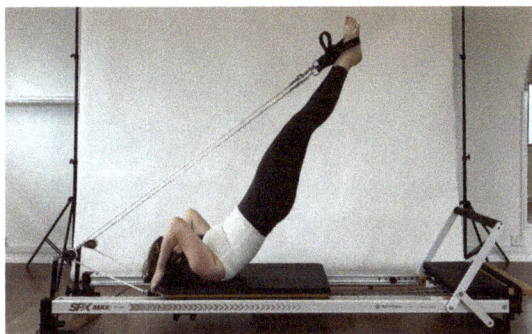

B
EXHALE

1. Extend both legs out to a 45 degree angle or challenge yourself to go slightly lower. Your spine remains elevated off the carriage.

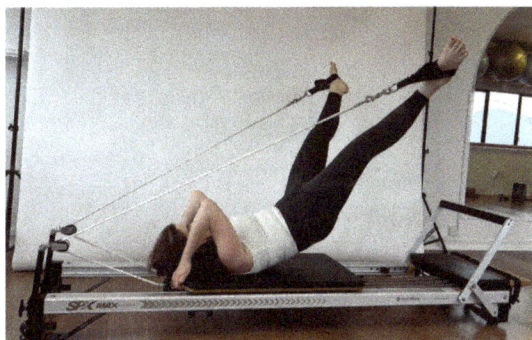

C
INHALE

1. Open your legs sideways.

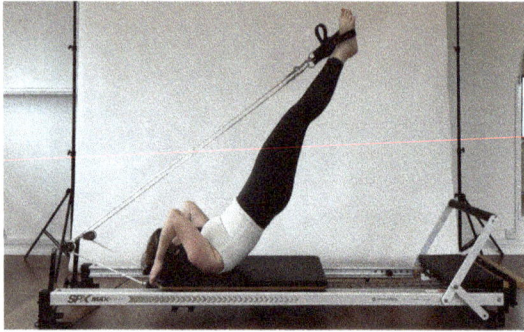

D

EXHALE

1. Close your legs.

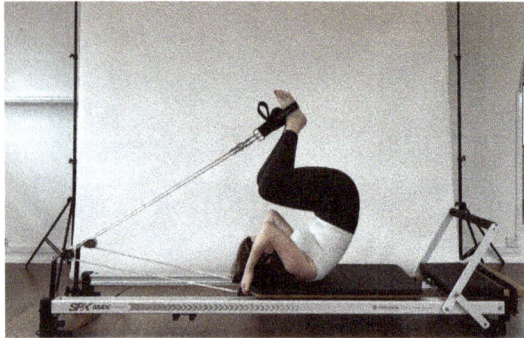

E

INHALE

1. Return to position **A**.

PROGRESSION 1

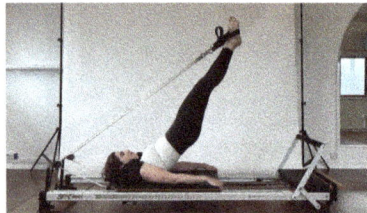

1. Place both arms on the carriage next to your body **(B)**

PROGRESSION 2

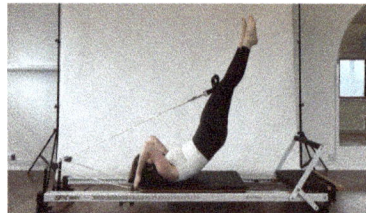

1. Both hands hold onto the back of the carriage and both knees in the straps **(B)**

PROGRESSION 3

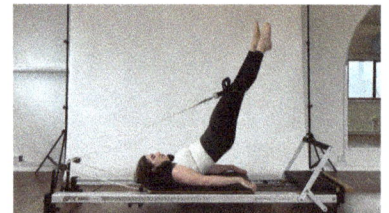

1. Place both arms on the carriage next to your body and both knees in the straps **(B)**

HUMAN FLAG I

Strength: Shoulders, arms, abs, glutes, hamstrings, inner thighs

Level: Advanced   **Repetition:** 8-10   **Springs:** Medium

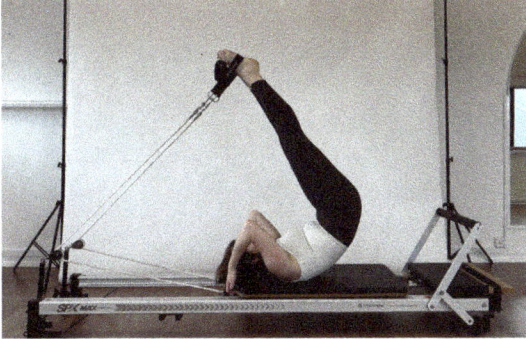

A
START

1. Hold onto the back of the carriage with both hands. Your elbows point up toward the ceiling.
2. Roll over onto your shoulder blades, extending your legs diagonally backward.

Intermediate: Both straps
Advance: Single strap

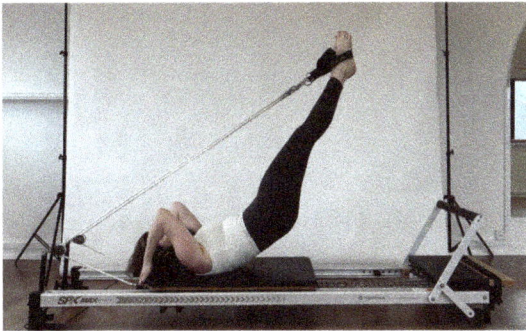

B
EXHALE

1. Extend both legs forward to a 45 degrees angle. Your spine remains lifted off the carriage.

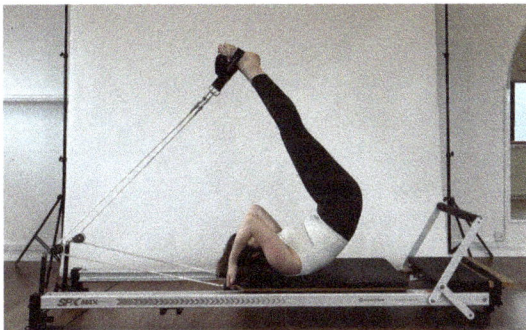

C
INHALE

1. Return to position **A**.

PROGRESSION 1

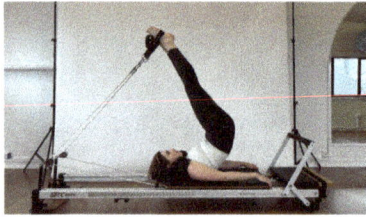

1. Place both arms on the carriage next to your body **(A)**

PROGRESSION 2

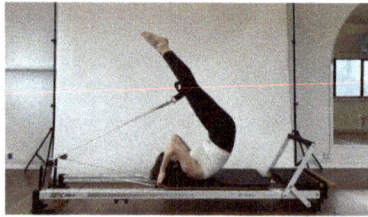

1. Both hands hold onto the back of the carriage and both knees are in the straps **(A)**

PROGRESSION 3

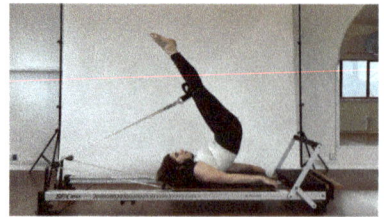

1. Place both arms on the carriage next to your body and both knees in the straps **(A)**

HUMAN FLAG II

Strength: Shoulder, arms, abs, glutes, hamstrings, inner thighs

Level: Advanced   **Repetition:** 8-10   **Springs:** Medium

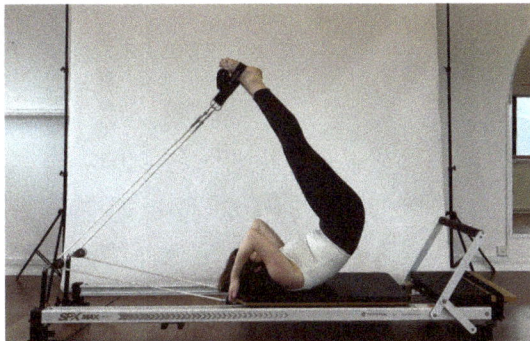

A
START

1. Hold onto the back of the carriage with both hands. Your elbows point up toward the ceiling
2. Roll over onto your shoulder blades, extending your legs diagonally backward.

Intermediate: Both straps
Advance: Single strap

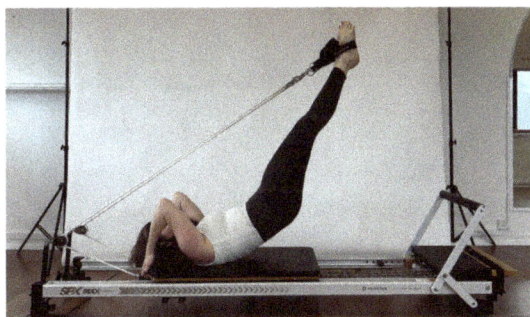

B
EXHALE

1. Extend both legs forward to a 45 degrees angle. Your spine remains lifted off the carriage.

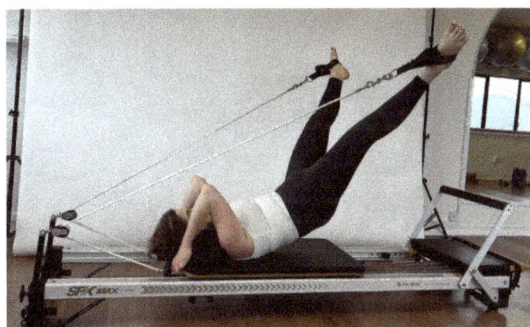

C
INHALE

1. Open your legs sideways.

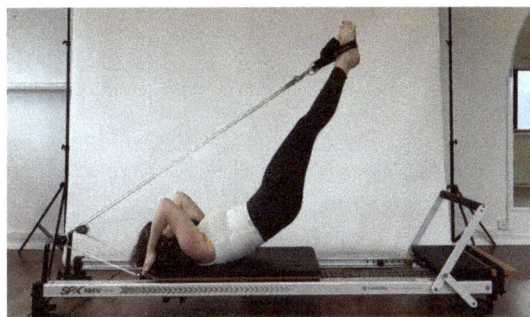

D
EXHALE

1. Close your legs

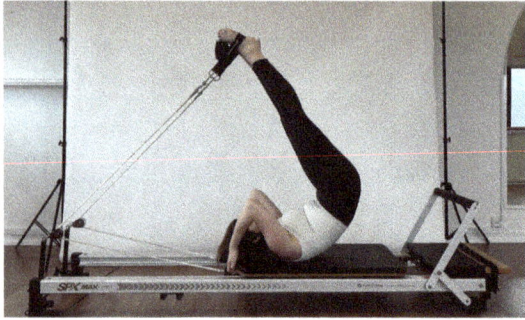

E

INHALE

1. Return to position **A**.

PROGRESSION 1

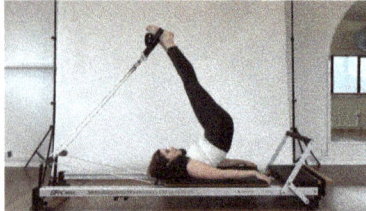

1. Place both arms on the carriage next to your body **(A)**

PROGRESSION 2

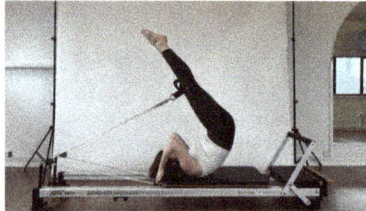

1. Both hands hold onto the back of the carriage and both knees in straps

PROGRESSION 3

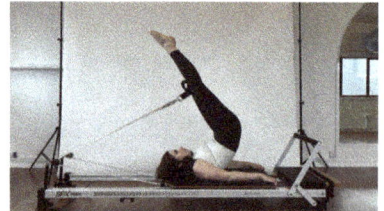

1. Arms on carriage, knees in straps **(A)**

RUNNING MAN I

Strength: Shoulder, arms, abs, bum, hamstring, inner thigh

Level: Advance   **Repetition:** 8-10   **Springs:** medium

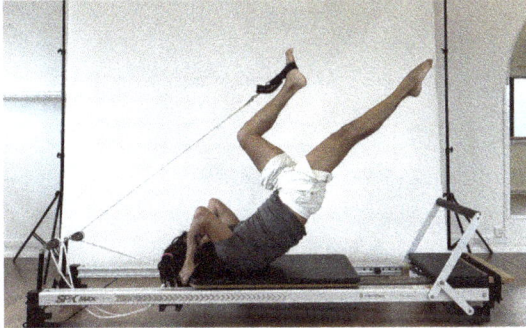

A
START

1. Place one foot in a strap. Bend the knee and extend the other strap free leg out in line with your hip.
2. Hold onto the back of the carriage. Your elbows point up toward the ceiling
3. Articulate your spine up to the middle of your upper spine.

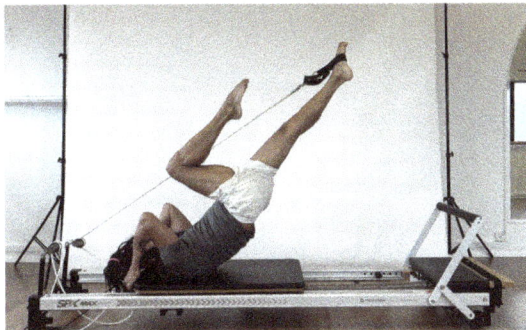

B
EXHALE

1. Swap legs, extending the strap leg and bending the free leg.

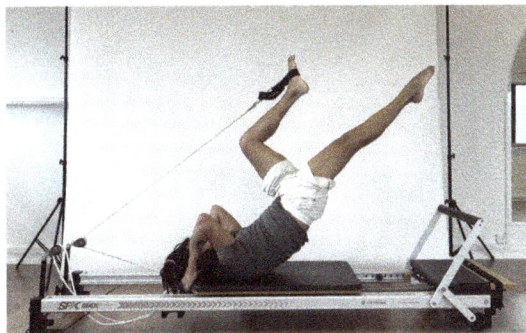

C
INHALE

1. Return to position **A**
2. Continue repeating the leg switches.

PROGRESSION 1

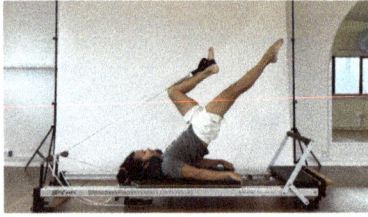

1. Place both arms next to your body on the carriage **(A)**

PROGRESSION 2

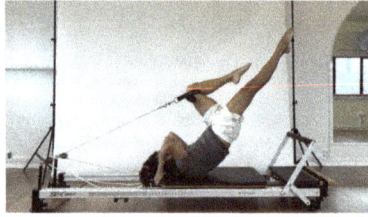

1. Hold onto the back of the carriage with both hands and place one knee in a strap **(A)**

PROGRESSION 3

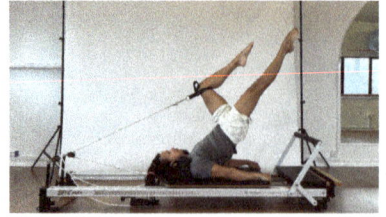

1. Place both arms next to your body on the carriage. Place one knee in a strap **(A)**

RUNNING MAN II

Strength: Shoulder, arms, abs, glutes, hamstrings, inner thighs

Level: Advanced   **Repetition:** 8-10   **Springs:** Medium

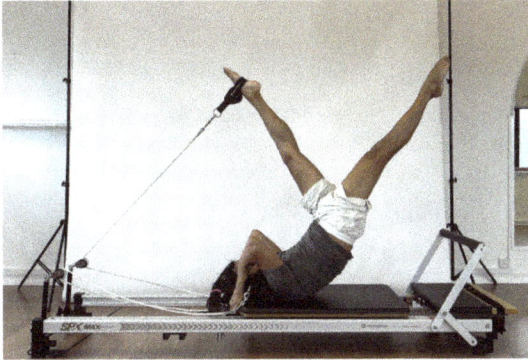

A
START

1. Hold onto the back of the carriage with both hands. Elbows point directly up toward the ceiling.
2. Place one foot in a strap and articulate your spine off the carriage.
3. Separate your legs with the strap leg coming toward you and the other leg extends forward to the wall in front of you.

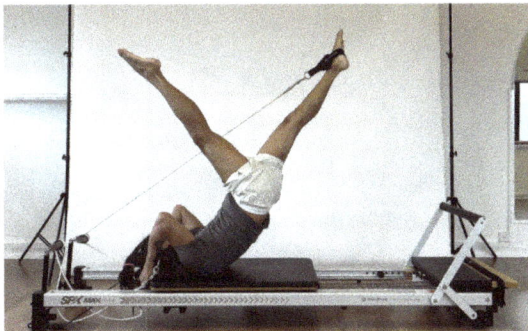

B
EXHALE

1. Swap the leg position. Your strap leg moves forward and the other leg scissors back toward you.

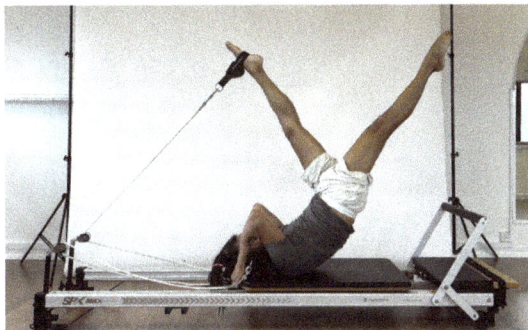

C
INHALE

1. Return to position **A**.
2. Continue repeating the scissor action.

PROGRESSION 1

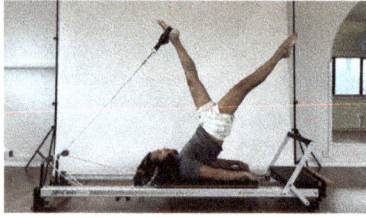

1. Place both arms next to your body on the carriage **(A)**

PROGRESSION 2

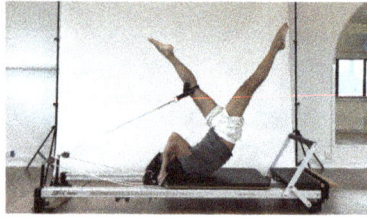

1. Hold onto the back of the carriage with both hands and place one knee in a strap **(A)**

PROGRESSION 3

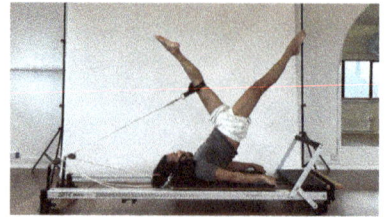

1. Place both arms next to your body on the carriage. Place one knee in a strap **(A)**

THE BOW I

Strength: Shoulder, arms, abs, glutes, hamstrings, inner thighs

Level: Advanced   **Repetition:** 8-10   **Springs:** Medium

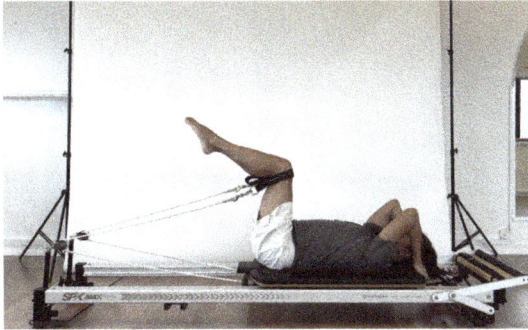

A
START

1. Lie on your back on the carriage with your head facing the footbar end.
2. Hold onto the edge of the carriage with both hands. Your elbows point up toward the ceiling.
3. Place your legs in table top position and the straps around your knees.

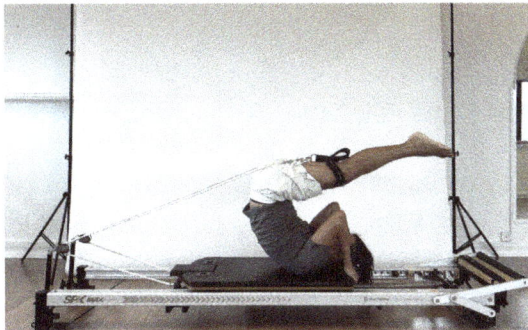

B
EXHALE

1. Roll over, bring your knees over your elbows and extend your legs to the wall behind you at the same time.

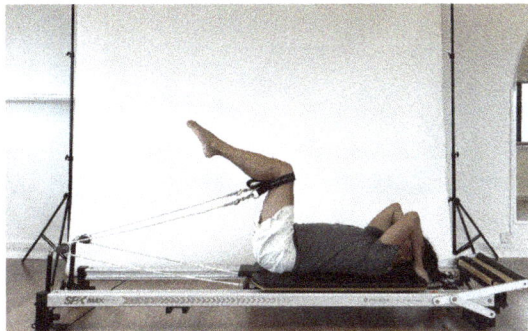

C
INHALE

1. Return to position **A**

THE BOW II

Strength: Shoulder, arms, abs, glutes, hamstrings, inner thighs

Level: Advanced   **Repetition:** 8-10   **Springs:** Medium

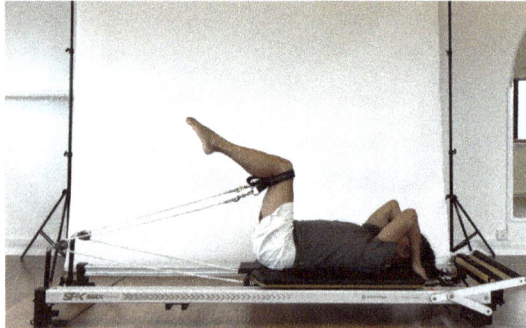

A

START

1. Lie on your back on the carriage with your head facing the footbar end.
2. Hold onto the edge of the carriage with both hands. Your elbows point up toward the ceiling.
3. Place your legs in table top position and the straps around your knees.

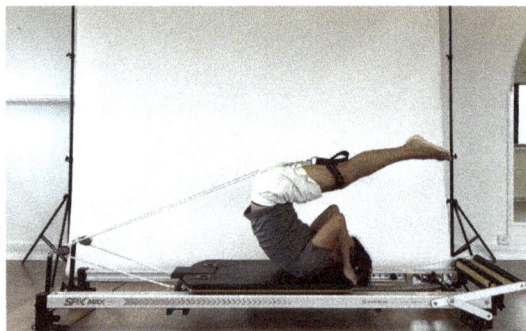

B

EXHALE

1. Roll over, bring your knees over your elbows and extend your legs to the wall behind you at the same time.

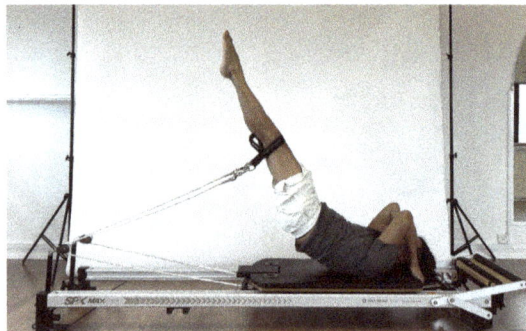

C

INHALE

1. Keep your spine elevated as you extend your legs away from your body until your feet point up toward the ceiling.
2. You can choose how you get to this position, try doing a circle or any variation you prefer.

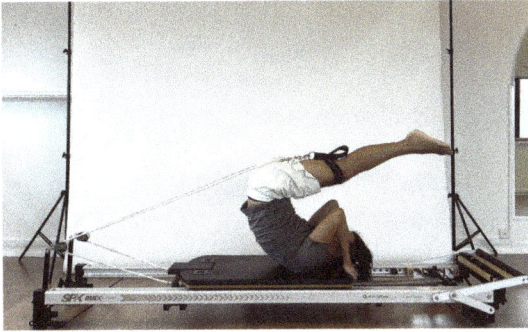

D
EXHALE

1. Return to position B

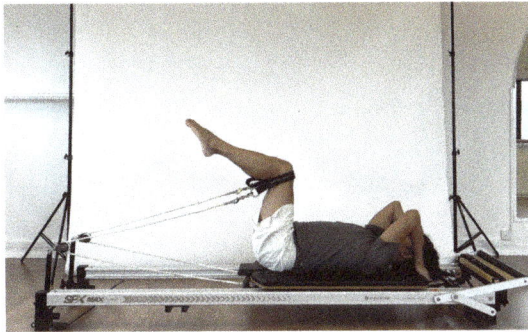

E
INHALE

1. Return to position **A**

PENDULUM

Strength: Abs, quads, inner thighs

Level: Intermediate   **Repetition:** 8-10   **Springs:** Medium

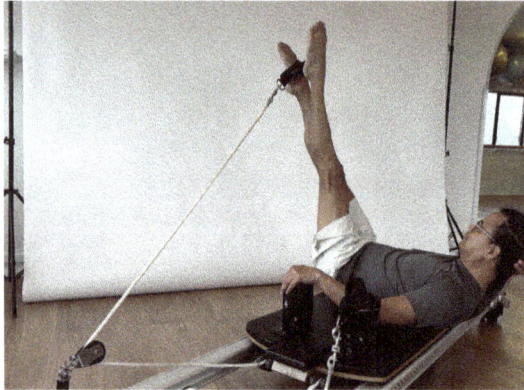

A
START

1. Lie sideways on the carriage on your back.
2. Place one arm against the shoulder rests and the other hand supports your head.
3. Place the strap on your footbar side foot. Extend both legs up toward the ceiling in a small V -heels touch, toes apart.

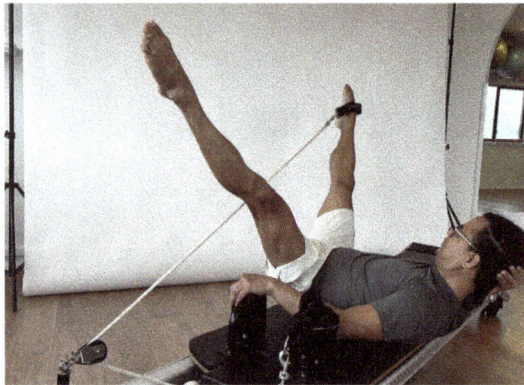

B

EXHALE

1. Open both legs away from each other

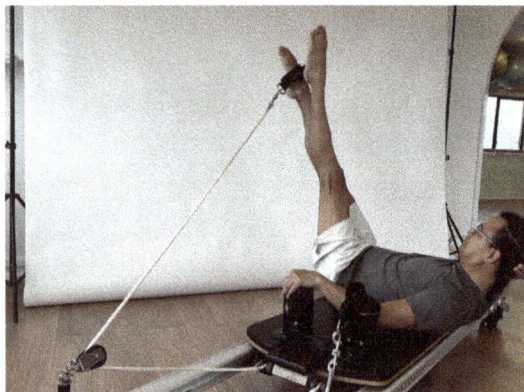

C

INHALE

1. Return to position **A**
2. Repeat with the strap on the other foot

PROGRESSION 1

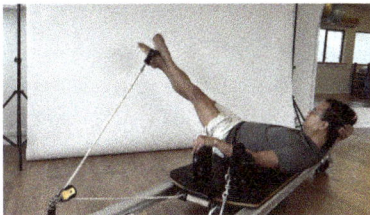

1. Extend both legs to 45 degrees **(A)**

PROGRESSION 2

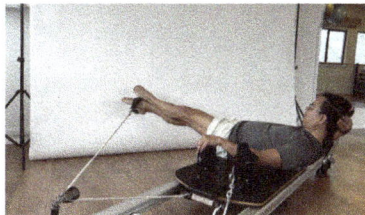

1. Extend both legs to 180 degrees **(A)**

ANCHOR I

Strength: Shoulder, arms, abs, glutes, hamstrings, inner thigh

Level: Advanced   **Repetition:** 8-10   **Springs:** Medium

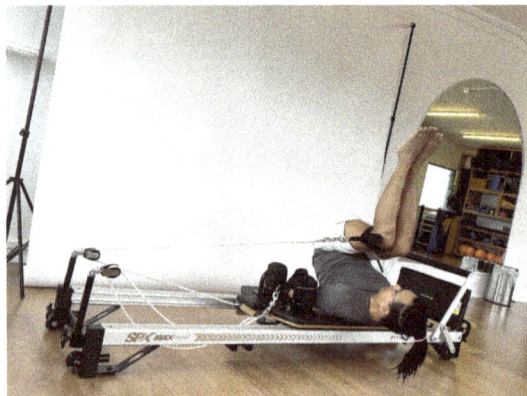

A
START

1. Lying sideways on the carriage on your back.
2. Your head is off the carriage
3. Place the strap around your knee closest to the shoulder rests.
4. Hold onto the side edge of the carriage with both hands.
5. Roll over bringing your knees above your shoulders. Bring the legs together.

Option: Place one foot in the strap

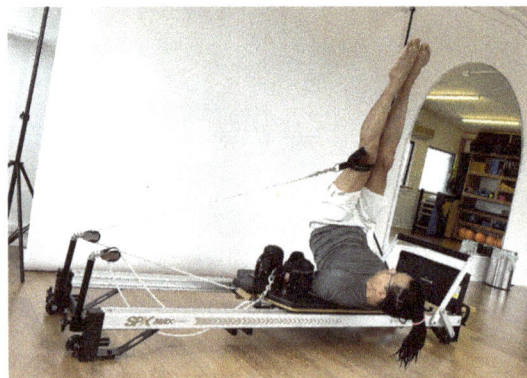

B
EXHALE

1. Extend your legs toward the ceiling.

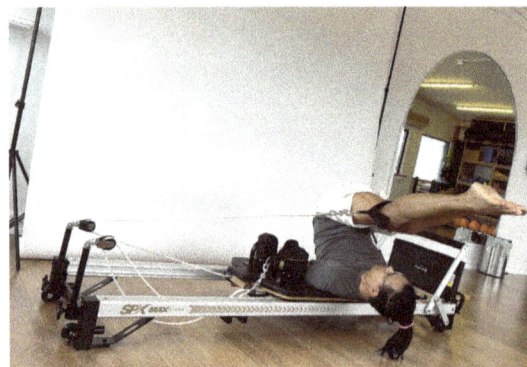

C
INHALE

1. Lower your legs towards the floor until they are parallel with the floor.

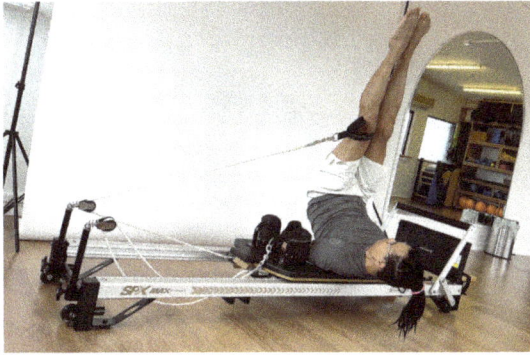

D

EXHALE

1. Return to position B

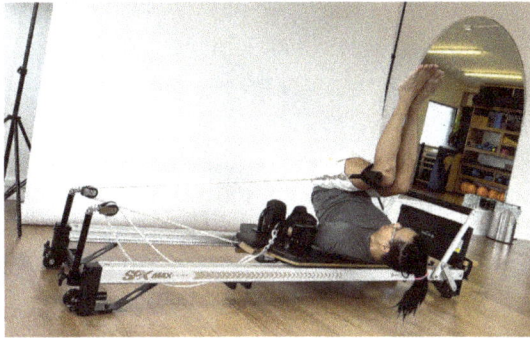

E

INHALE

1. Return to position **A**.
2. Repeat on the other side.

ANCHOR II

Strength: Shoulders, arms, abs, glutes, hamstrings, inner thighs

Level: Advanced　　　　**Repetition:** 8-10　　　　**Springs:** Medium

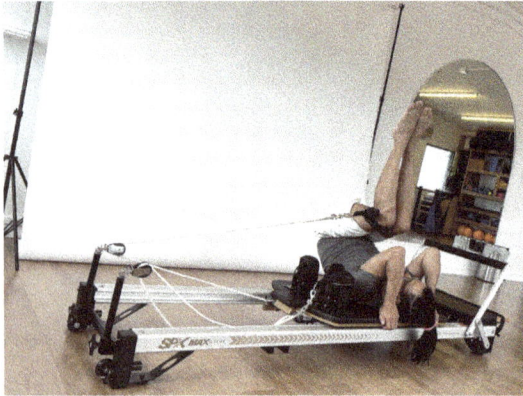

A
START

1. Lie sideways across the carriage on your back. Your head is on the carriage.
2. Hold onto the side edge of the carriage with both hands. Your elbows point straight up toward the ceiling.
3. Roll over with bent knees until your knees are over your elbows. Bring your knees together.
4. Place one strap on the knee closest to the shoulder rest.

Option: Place one foot in the strap.

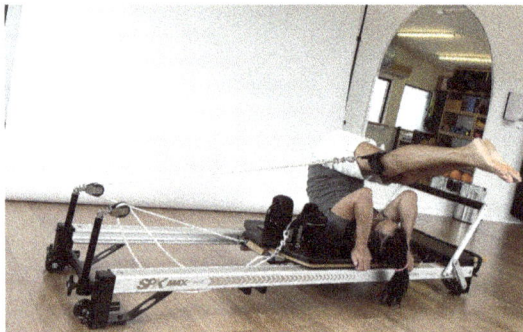

B
EXHALE

1. Extend your legs so they are parallel with the floor.

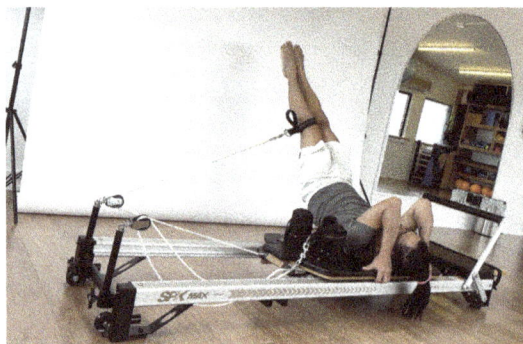

C
INHALE

1. Bring your legs forward to a 45 degree angle keeping your spine elevated.

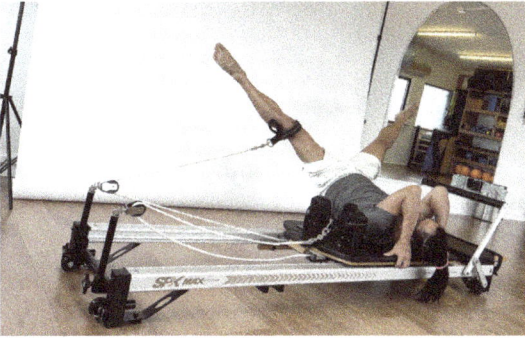

D

EXHALE

1. Open and close your legs.

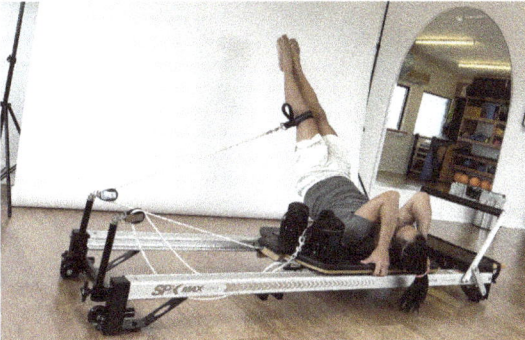

E

INHALE

1. Briefly hold position **C.**

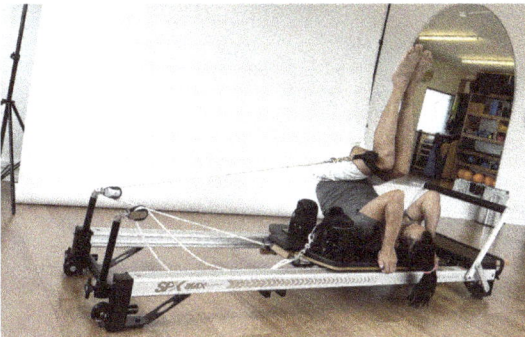

F

EXHALE

1. 1 Return to position **A**.
2. Repeat on the other side.

UNTOLD
PART IV

ROCKET LAUNCHER

Strength: Glutes, hamstrings, quads, calves

Level: Intermediate   **Repetition:** 8-10   **Springs:** Light to medium

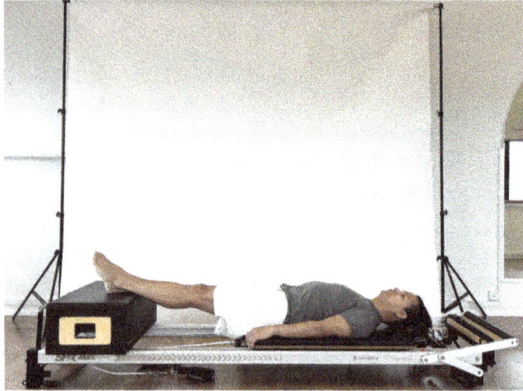

A
START

1. Lie on your back with your head toward the footbar end.
2. Hold onto the end of the carriage with both hands firmly.
3. Place your heels on top of the reformer box. The box is placed at the riser end of the reformer across the frame.
4. Flex your ankles and place your legs together. Separate your feet if you feel tension in your lower back.
5. Remove the shoulder rests if possible.

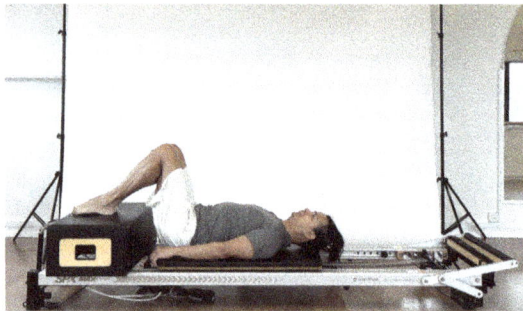

B
EXHALE

1. Press heels down and bend your knees bringing the carriage toward the box.

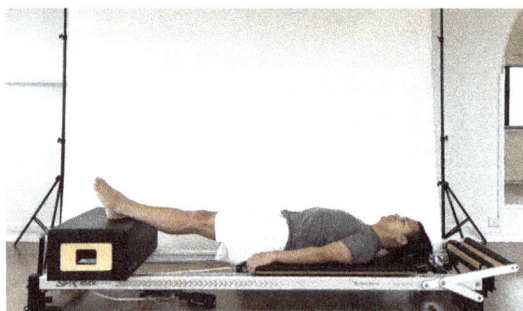

C
INHALE

1. Return to position **A**.

PROGRESSION 1

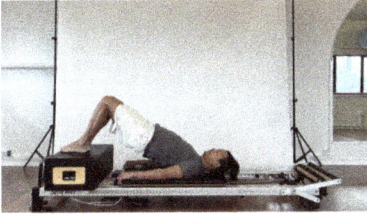

1. Lift your hips as you bring the carriage toward the box **(B)**

PROGRESSION 2

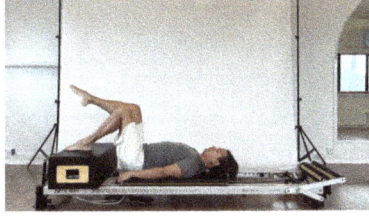

1. Do a single leg bend. The other leg is in table top and the hips are on the carriage **(B)**

PROGRESSION 3

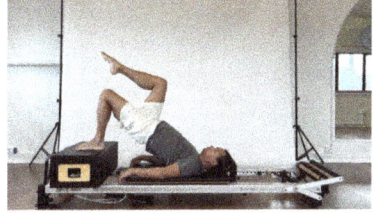

1. Lift your hips and one leg into the air. **(B)**

ICE SKATER I

Strength: Shoulders, oblique, glutes, quads, hamstrings

Level: Intermediate   **Repetition:** 8-10   **Springs:** Medium

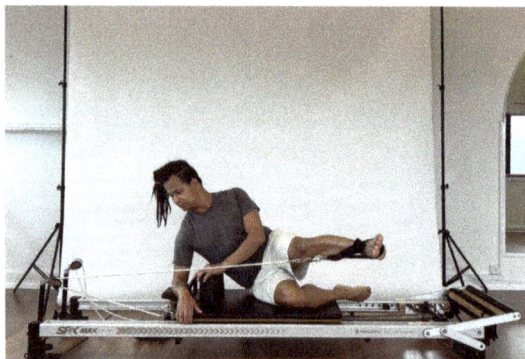

A

START

1. Face sideways and place your body in a half side plank position with your knees bent at 90 degrees in front of you.
2. Place your elbow on top of the headrest
3. Place the other hand on top of the shoulder rest in front of you.
4. Place your top foot in the strap and extend the leg out in front of you.

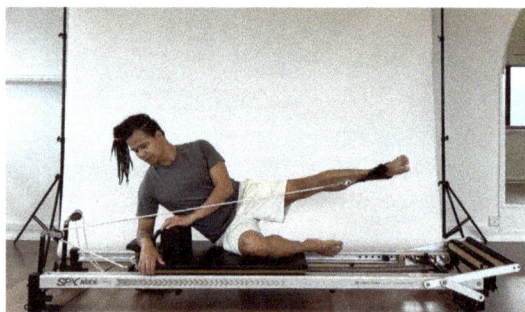

B

EXHALE

1. Arc your strap leg backward into extension.
2. Keep your leg at the same height as your hip.

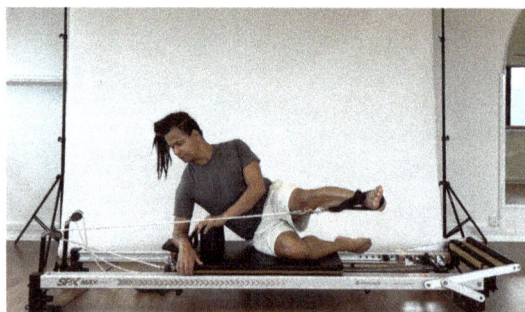

C

INHALE

1. Return to position **A**.
2. Repeat on the other side.

PROGRESSION 1

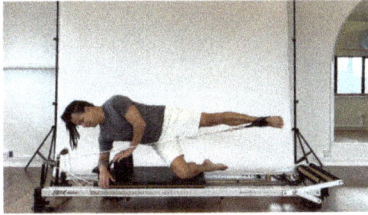

1. Kneeling side plank **(B)**

PROGRESSION 2

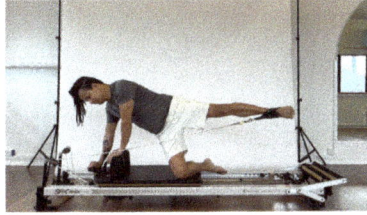

1. Extend your arm. Place your hand on the headrest and body in a kneeling side plank **(B)**

PROGRESSION 3

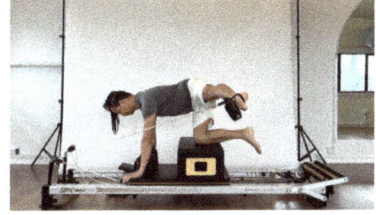

1. Kneel on top of the reformer box. Place your hands beside the shoulder rests. Your trunk faces the carriage. Place the strap on one leg and extend it out sideways from your hip **(A)**

PROGRESSION 4

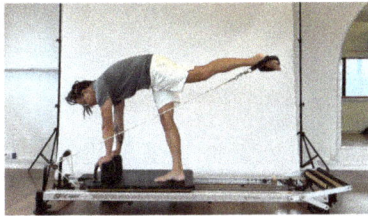

1. As for progression 3 but remove the box and stand on the reformer carriage. Place your hands on the shoulder rests **(A)**

ICE SKATER II

Strength: Shoulders, obliques, quads, glutes, hamstrings

Level: Intermediate　　　**Repetition:** 8-10　　　**Springs:** Medium

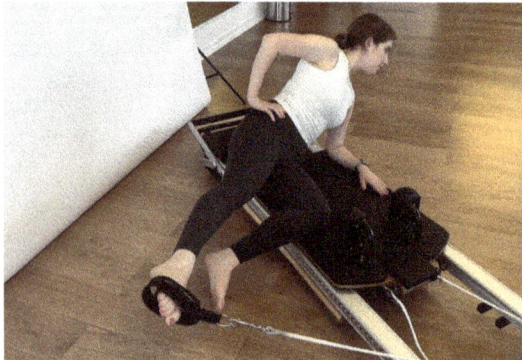

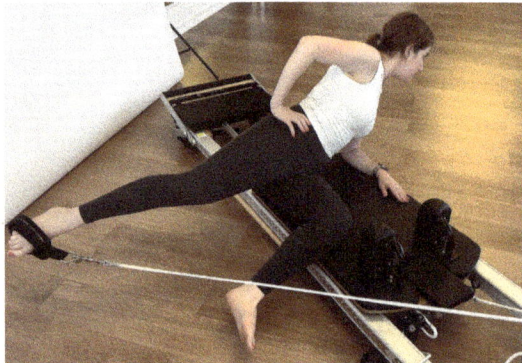

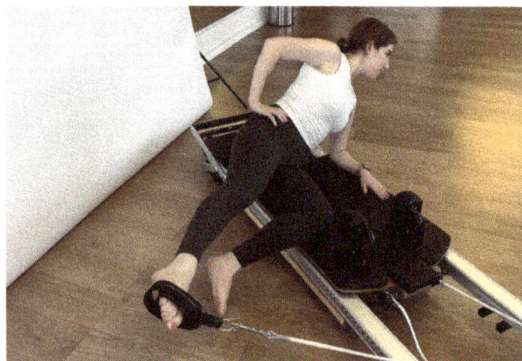

A
START

1. Side sitting position with your forearm. supporting you. Place the forearm on the bottom edge of the reformer carriage.
2. Line your hips up along the edge of the reformer carriage in line with your arm. Your lower knee is bent.
3. Place your upper hand on your hips.
4. Place your top foot in the strap.

B
EXHALE

1. Swing your strap leg backward towards the footbar.
2. Keep your leg at the same height as your upper hip.

C
INHALE

1. Return to position **A**
2. Repeat on the other side

REVERSE ICE SKATER

Strength: Abs, quads, glutes, hamstrings

Level: Intermediate   **Repetition:** 8-10   **Springs:** Medium

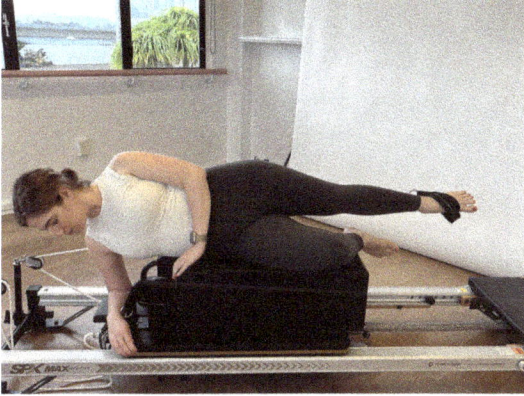

A
START

1. Place the reformer box on the carriage in the long box position.
2. Lie on your side in the middle of the box. Place the lower forearm across the headrest and your upper hand in front of you on the box.
3. Place your upper leg's foot in the strap and extend the leg at hip height in line with your spine.
4. Bend the lower leg to create more support for your body on the box.

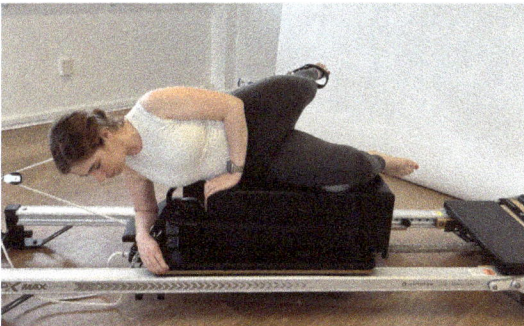

B
EXHALE

1. Swing your upper leg behind you, extending your hip. Support your lumbar spine with your abdominals to protect your lower back.

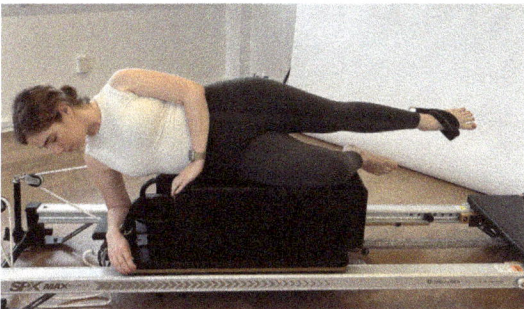

C
INHALE

1. Return to position **A**.
2. Repeat on the other side.

PEDAL PUSHER I

Strength: Chest, shoulders, abs, quads, glutes, hamstrings

Level: Intermediate   **Repetition:** 8-10   **Springs:** Light to medium

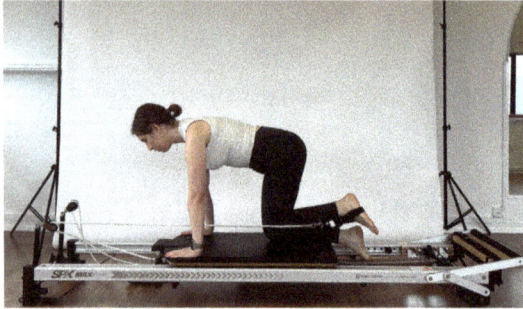

A
START

1. Kneel on the carriage toward the footbar end of the reformer. Place one strap on one foot.
2. Place your hands on the upper edge of the carriage in four point kneel. Make sure the rope runs between your arm.

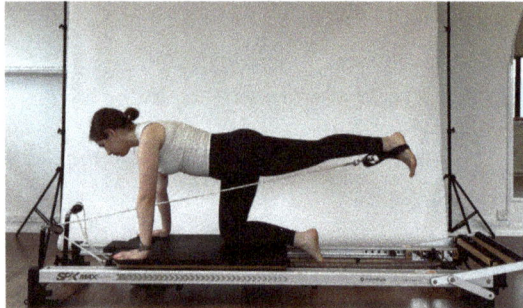

B
EXHALE

1. Extend the strap leg backward using your glutes and hamstrings.

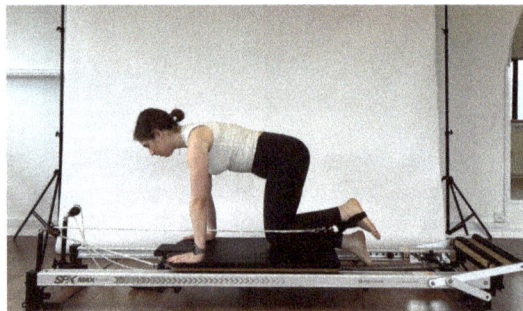

C
INHALE

1. Return to position **A**.
2. Repeat on the other side.

PEDAL PUSHER II

Strength: Chest, shoulders, abs, quads, glutes, hamstrings

Level: Intermediate   **Repetition:** 8-10   **Springs:** Light to medium

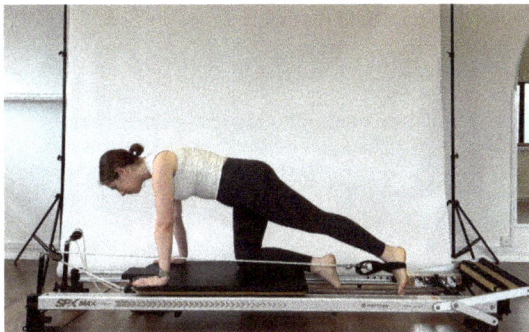

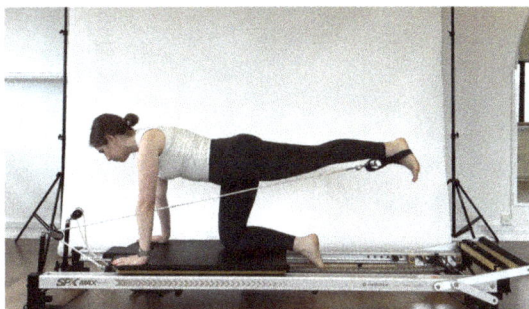

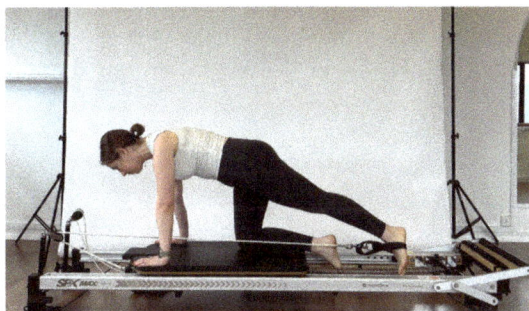

A
START

1. Kneel on the carriage toward the footbar end of the reformer. Place one strap on one foot and extend that leg with the foot in the well of the reformer..
2. Place your hands on the upper edge of the carriage in four point kneel. Make sure the rope runs between your arm.

B
EXHALE

1. Lift your extended leg up as high as you can while maintaining your spinal alignment.

C
INHALE

1. Return to position **A**
2. Repeat on the other side.

PROGRESSION 1

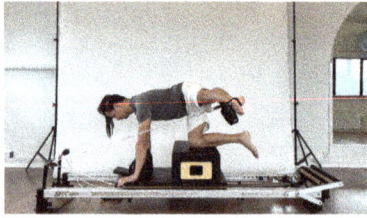

1. Kneel on top of the box. Place your hands at the top edge of the carriage and extend the strap leg out toward the side. Make sure the strap is on the outside of your arm. **(B)**

PROGRESSION 2

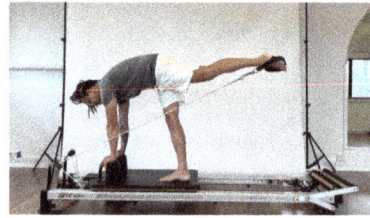

1. Stand on the reformer with the strap on the extended leg - Elephant arabesque position. Place your hands on the shoulder rests and the strap on the outside of your arm. **(B)**

NOSE DIVE I

Strength: Chest, shoulders, abs, glutes, hamstrings

Level: Intermediate   **Repetition:** 8-10   **Springs:** Light to medium

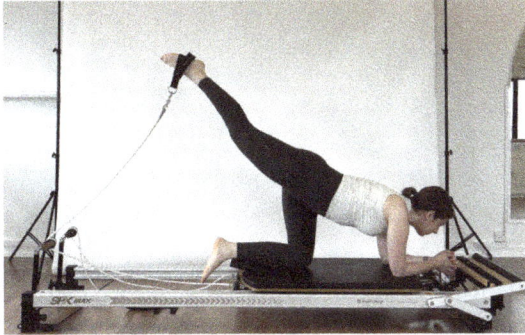

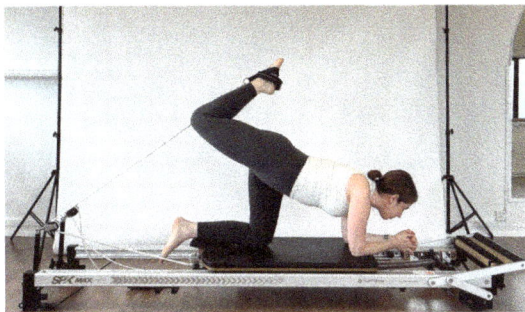

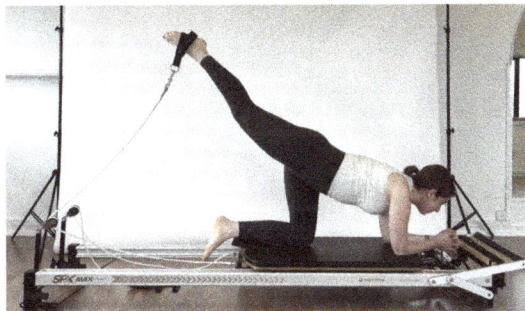

A
START

1. Four point kneeling facing the footbar end. Your forearms are on the carriage and one strap is placed on one foot. Extend the leg behind and upward in line with your hip.
2. Keep the rope tension tight in the starting position.

B
EXHALE

1. Bend your knee, pulling your heel to your hip. Keep the knee in the same place, don't drop it.

C
INHALE

1. Return to position **A**.
2. Repeat on the other side.

PROGRESSION 1

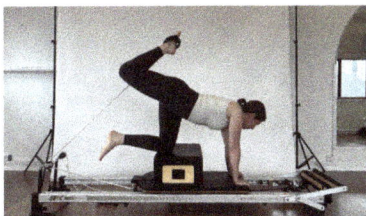

1. Kneel on top of the box. Place your hands on the carriage. **(B)**

PROGRESSION 2

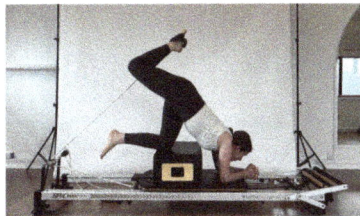

1. Kneel on top of the box and place your forearms on the carriage **(B)**

NOSE DIVE II

Strength: Chest, shoulders, abs, glutes, hamstrings

Level: Intermediate   **Repetition:** 8-10   **Springs:** Light to medium

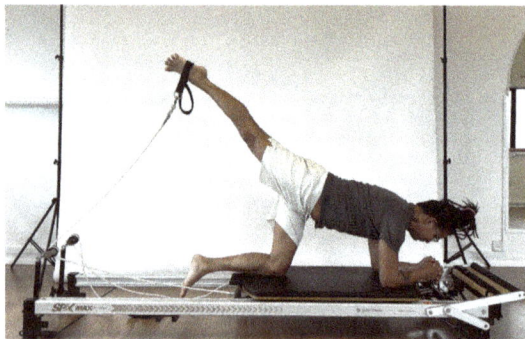

A
START

1. Four point kneeling facing the footbar end. Your forearms are on the carriage and one strap is placed on one foot. Extend the leg behind and upward in line with your hip.
2. Keep the rope tension tight in the starting position.

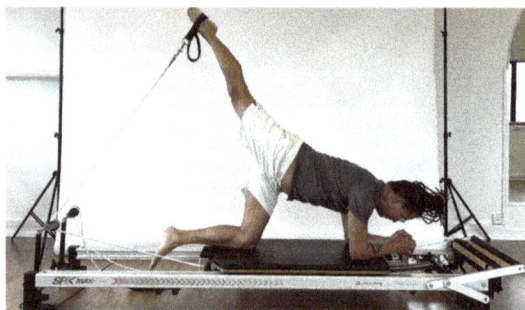

B
EXHALE

1. Lift your strap leg up to the ceiling.

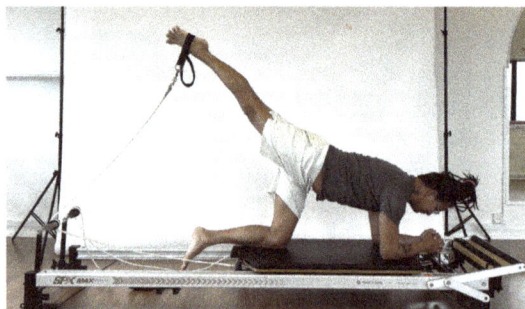

C
INHALE

1. Return to position **A**
2. Repeat on the other side

PROGRESSION 1

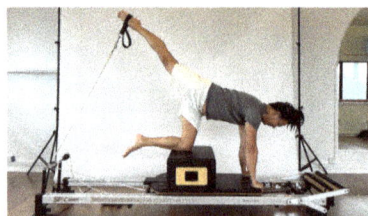

1. Kneel on top of the box and your hands on the carriage **(B)**

PROGRESSION 2

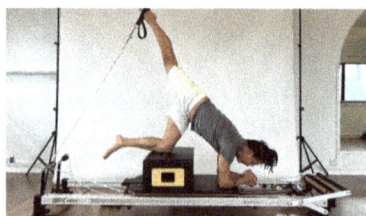

1. Kneel on the reformer box and place your forearms on the carriage **(B)**

SIDE SLIDE I

Strength: Chest, shoulders, arms, abs, obliques, glutes, hamstrings, inner thigh

Level: Intermediate   **Repetition:** 8-10   **Springs:** Light to medium

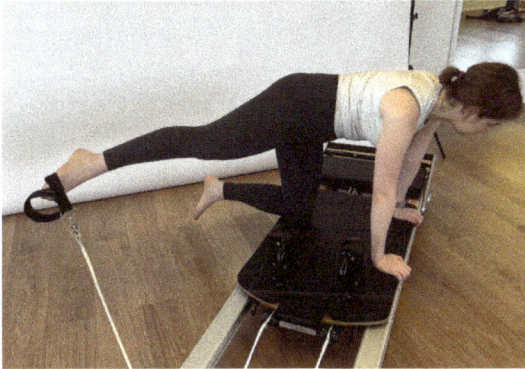

A
START

1. Four point kneeling across the carriage sideways. Your hands hold onto the edge of the reformer.
2. Place a strap on the leg closest to the shoulder rests. Extend your leg behind you in line with your hip.
3. Keep the rope tight.

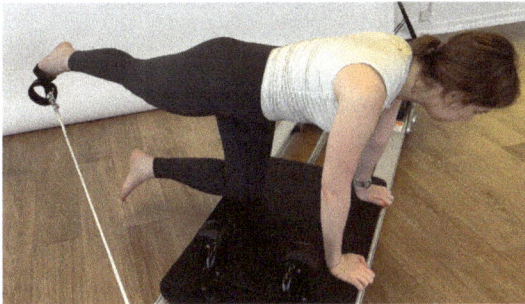

B
EXHALE

1. Pull your strap leg toward the footbar. You will do a small side bend of your spine shortening the side closest to the footbar.

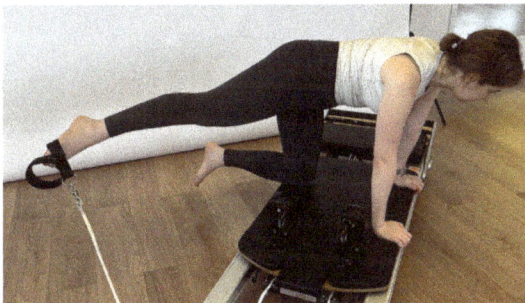

C
INHALE

1. Return to position **A**
2. Repeat on the other side.

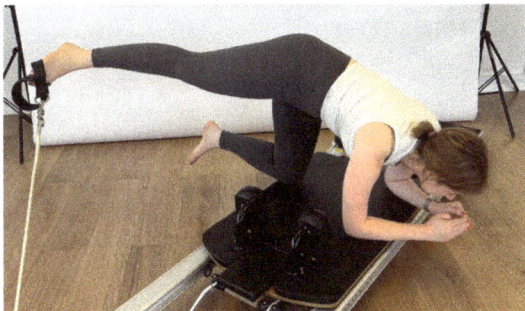

MODIFICATION

1. Place your elbows on the carriage.

SIDE SLIDE II

Strength: Chest, shoulders, arms, abs, obliques, glutes, hamstrings

Level: Intermediate **Repetition:** 8-10 **Springs:** Light to medium

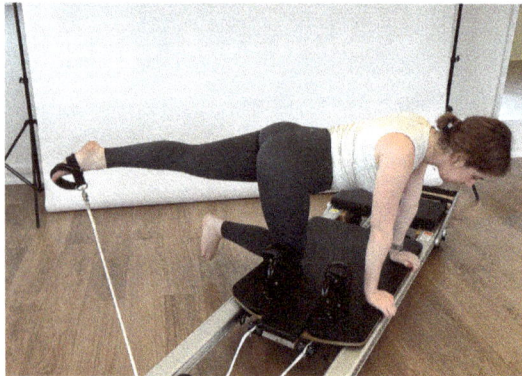

A
START

1. Four point kneeling across the carriage sideways. Your hands hold onto the edge of the reformer.
2. Place a strap on the leg closest to the footbar. Extend your leg behind you in line with your hip.
3. Keep the rope tight.

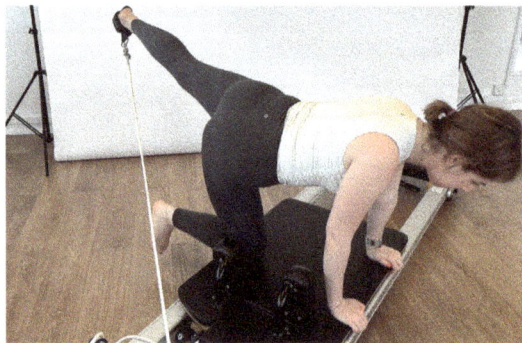

B
EXHALE

1. Pull your inner leg toward the footbar. You will side bend toward the shoulder rests as the leg moves across midline.

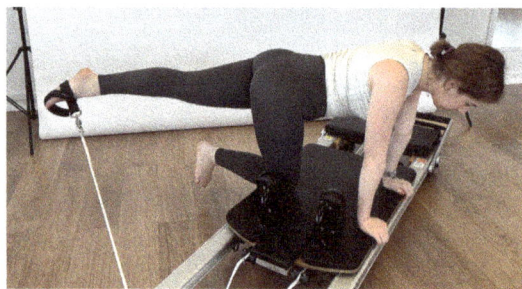

C
INHALE

1. Return to position **A**
2. Repeat on the other side

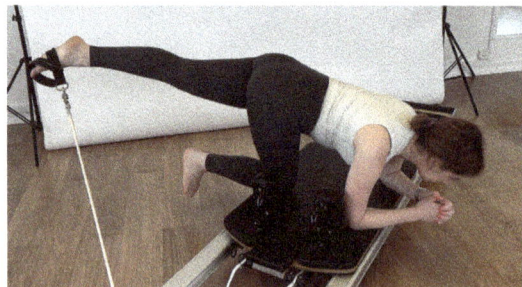

MODIFICATION

1. Place your elbows on the carriage.

SIDE SWIPE I

Strength: Chest, shoulders, arms, abs, oblique, glutes, hamstrings

Level: Intermediate   **Repetition:** 8-10   **Springs:** Light to medium

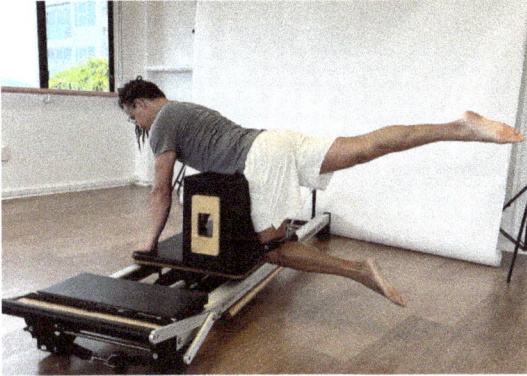

A
START

1. Stand next to the reformer facing the carriage. Place the reformer box in the long box position. The box is on its side toward the edge of the carriage closest to you
2. Place the strap on the footbar leg's knee. Place your pelvis on top of the box and hands on the other side at the edge of the carriage like a supported four point kneel.
3. Lift your riser end leg up behind you to hip height extending the knee.

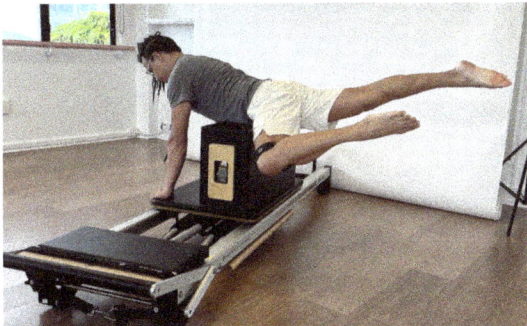

B
EXHALE

1. Open your bent knee sideways and up toward the footbar.

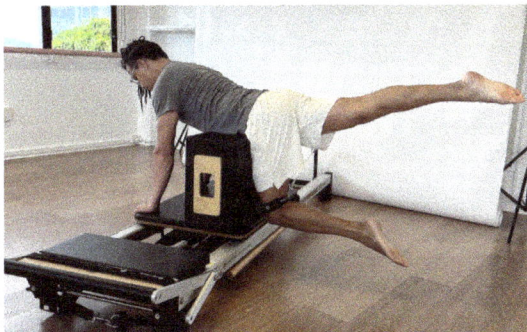

C
INHALE

1. Return to position **A**.
2. Repeat on the other side.

SIDE SWIPE II

Strength: Chest, shoulders, arms, abs, obliques, glutes, hamstrings

Level: Intermediate   **Repetition:** 8-10   **Springs:** Light to medium

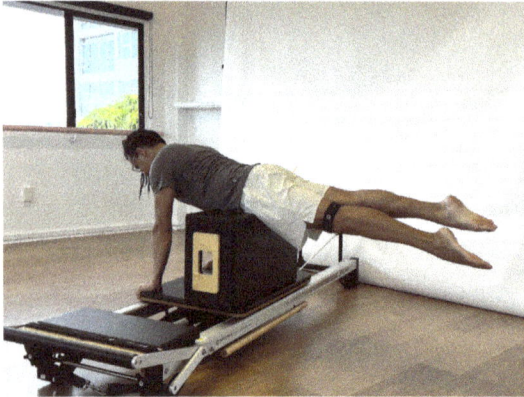

A
START

1. Stand next to the reformer facing the carriage. Place the reformer box in the long box position. The box is on its side toward the edge of the carriage closest to you.
2. Place the strap on the footbar leg's knee. Place your pelvis on top of the box and hands on the other side at the edge of the carriage like a supported four point kneel.
3. Lift both your legs up, extending them behind you.

Option: Place your foot in the strap

B
EXHALE

1. Open both legs away from each other

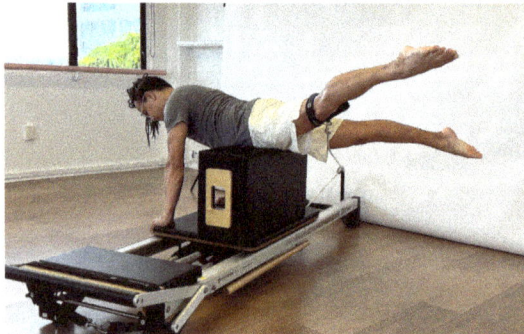

C
INHALE

1. Return to position **A**.
2. Repeat on the other side.

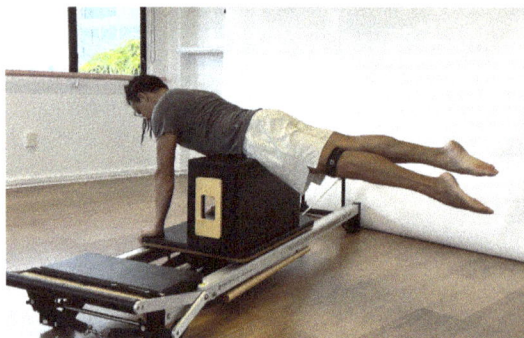

DEEP DIVE I

Strength: Chest, shoulders, abs, quads, glutes, hamstrings

Level: Intermediate   **Repetition:** 8-10   **Springs:** Light to medium

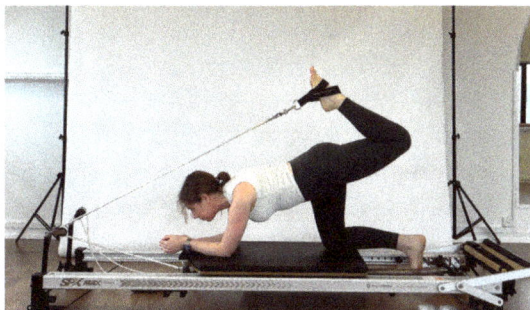

A
START

1. Four point kneeling on your forearms facing the riser end of the reformer.
2. Elbow on the carriage, hands at the edge
3. Place one foot in the strap. Bend your knee and bring your heel toward your bottom.

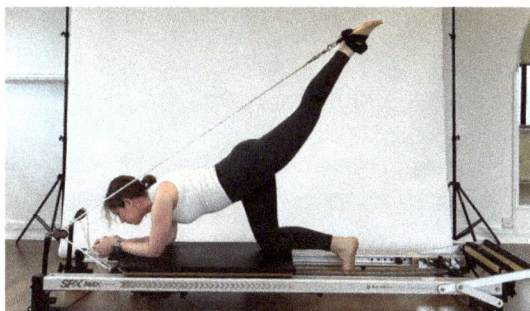

B
EXHALE

1. Extend your knee without dropping your leg.

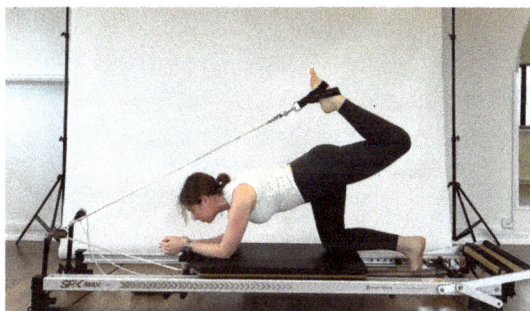

C
INHALE

1. Return to position **A**.
2. Repeat on the other side.

DEEP DIVE II

Strength: Chest, shoulder, abs, quads, glutes, hamstrings

Level: Intermediate   **Repetition:** 8-10   **Springs:** Light to medium

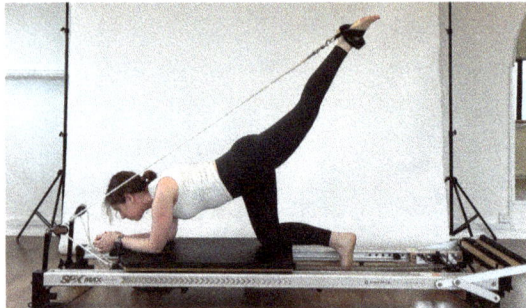

A
START

1. Four point kneeling on your forearms facing the riser end of the reformer.
2. Elbow on the carriage, hands at the edge
3. Place one foot in the strap. Extend your leg out behind you diagonally up toward the ceiling.

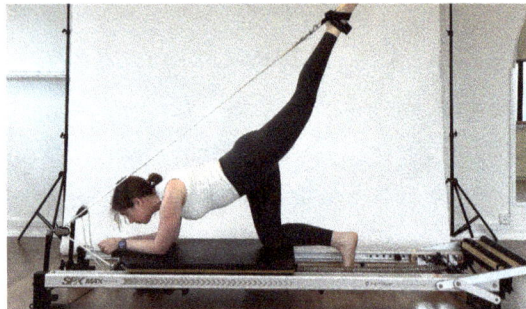

B
EXHALE

1. Lift your leg higher towards the ceiling.

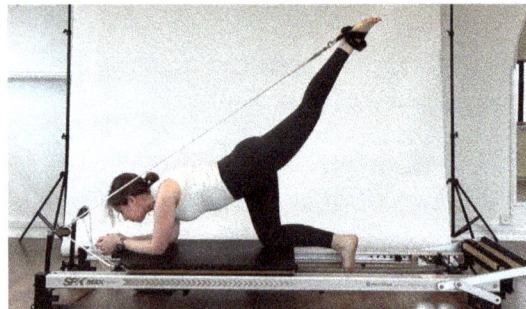

C
INHALE

1. Return to position **A**
2. Repeat on the other side

UNTOLD
PART V

CHOO CHOO TRAIN

Strength: Tricep, oblique, quads, glutes, inner thighs

Level: Intermediate   **Repetition:** 8-10   **Springs:** Light to medium

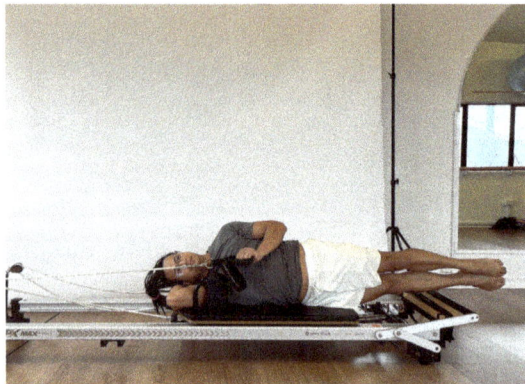

A
START

1. Lie sideways on the carriage with your legs extended in line with your spine. The footbar is down to make room for your legs. Support your head with your underneath arm and hand. Hold onto the shoulder rest with the underneath hand.
2. The upper hand holds the strap, elbow bent on top of the rib cage.
3. Slightly lift both legs off.

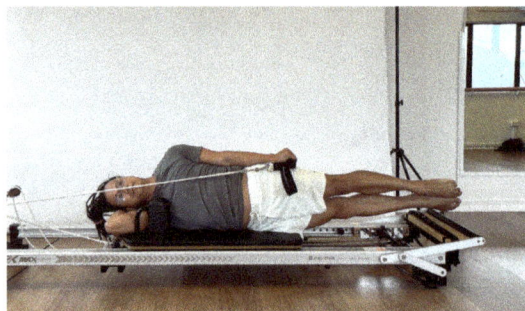

B
EXHALE

1. Extend your elbow pulling the strap down toward your feet.

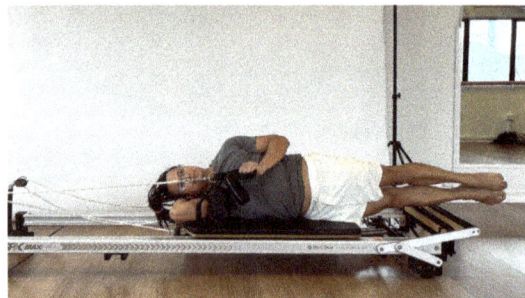

C
INHALE

1. Return to position **A**.
2. Repeat on the other side.

PROGRESSION 1

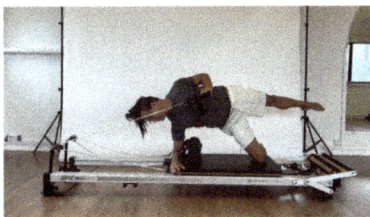

1. Advanced kneeling side kick position on your forearm. Hold onto the strap with your upper arm lying along the top of your ribs **(A)**

PROGRESSION 2

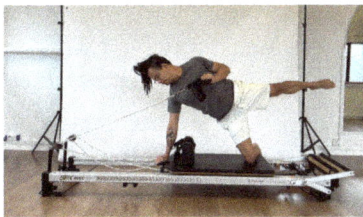

1. Advanced side kick position with the top hand holding onto the strap. Place your upper arm along the top of your ribs **(A)**

SPEAR HUNTER I

Strength: Arms, Abs

Level: Intermediate   **Repetition:** 8-10   **Springs:** Light to medium

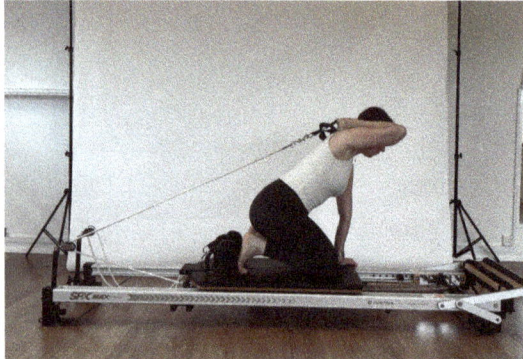

A
START

1. Face the footbar Japanese kneel in the toe tucked position against the shoulder rests.
2. One hand holds the strap. Bend your elbow and bring your hand behind your head. The elbow points forward
3. Hinge forward from your hips to place the other hand on the carriage in front of your knee.

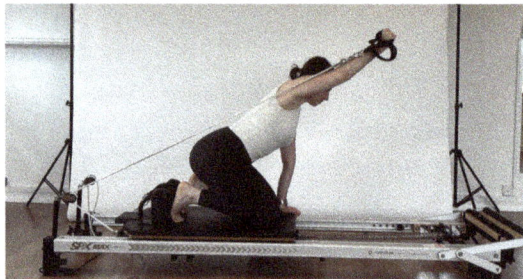

B
EXHALE

1. Extend your elbow, pulling the strap forward. Keep the upper arm where it is as you extend the elbow.

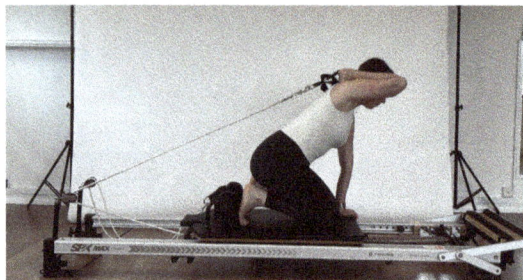

C
INHALE

1. Return to position **A**.
2. Repeat on the other side.

PROGRESSION 1

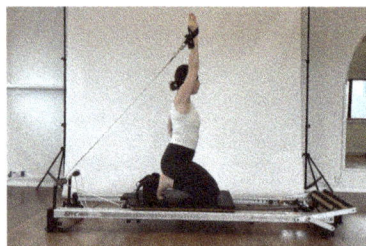

1. Sit upright on your heels in the Japanese kneeling position **(A)**

PROGRESSION 2

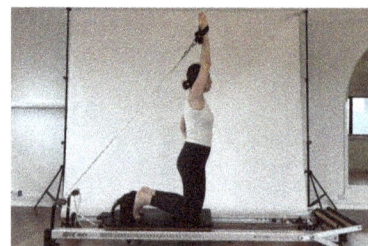

1. High kneel **(A)**

SPEAR HUNTER II

Strength: Arms, abs

Level: Intermediate   **Repetition:** 8-10   **Springs:** Light to medium

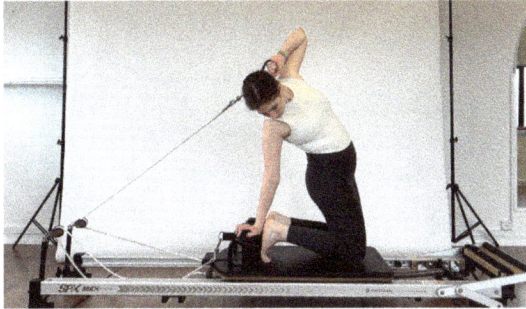

A
START

1. High kneel facing the footbar. Place one hand on the shoulder pad behind you. Hold the strap with the other hand behind your head
2. Clip your elbow in and facing up to ceiling
3. Press your feet against the shoulder rests.

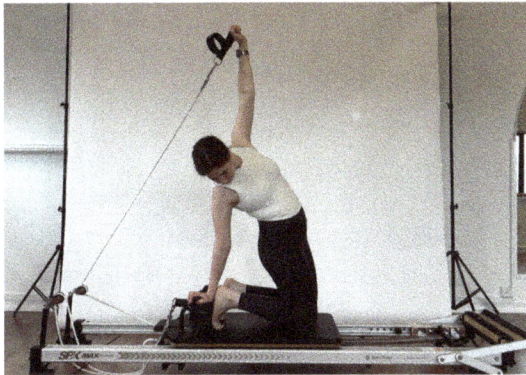

B
EXHALE

1. Extend your elbow without dropping your upper arm toward the floor.

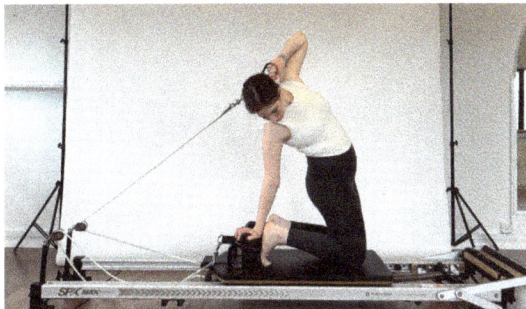

C
INHALE

1. Return to position **A**.
2. Repeat on the other side.

RIB OF ADAM I

Strength: Shoulder, tricep, oblique

Level: Intermediate   **Repetition:** 8-10   **Springs:** Light to medium

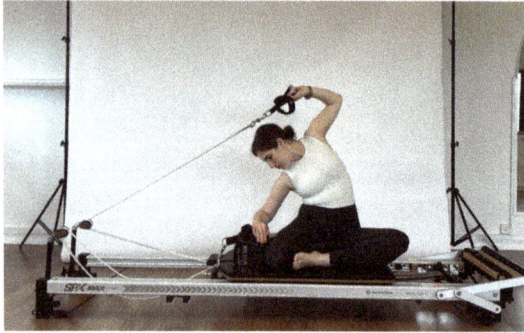

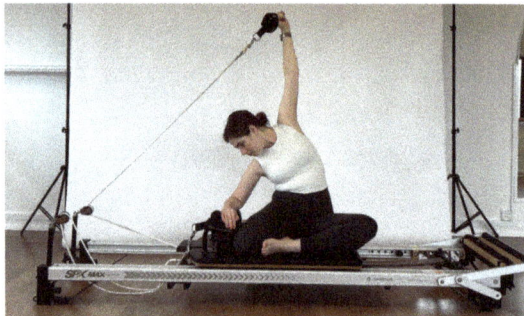

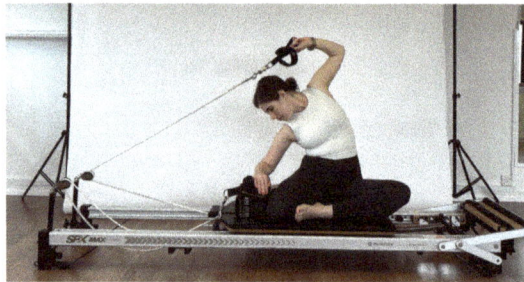

A

START

1. Place your legs in the Mermaid position and side bend toward the shoulder rests.
2. Place your forearm along the top of the
3. shoulder rests.
4. Bring the upper arm overhead and hold onto one strap. Your elbow points up toward the ceiling with your elbow bent.

B

EXHALE

1. Pull the strap straightening your elbow and your hand reaches up to the ceiling.

C

INHALE

1. Return to position **A**
2. Repeat on the other side

PROGRESSION 1

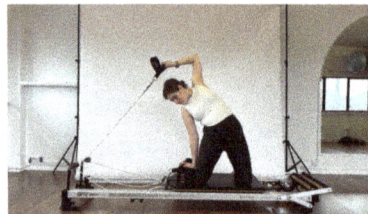

1. High kneel **(A)**

PROGRESSION 2

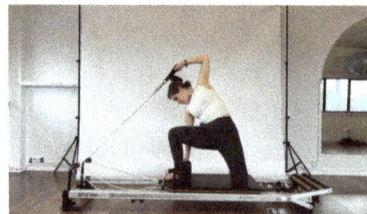

1. Kneel placing one foot on the headrest and lunge slightly sideways into the side bend **(A)**

PROGRESSION 3

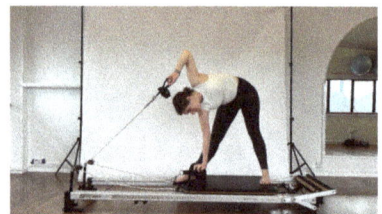

1. Stand on the carriage. Bend one leg and place the other foot on the headrest with the leg extended **(A)**

RIB OF ADAM II

Strength: Shoulder, tricep, obliques

Level: Intermediate   **Repetition:** 8-10   **Springs:** Light to medium

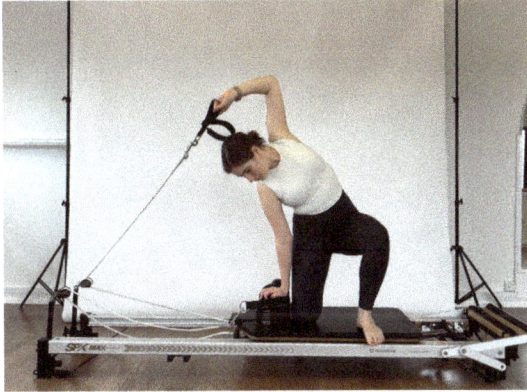

A
START

1. Kneel on the carriage with one leg below your hip. The leg closest to the footbar is extended forward and the foot is on the carriage. The knee is bent at 90 degrees.
2. Place your hand onto the shoulder rest and side bend toward that hand.
3. Bring the upper arm overhead and hold onto one strap. Your elbow points up toward the ceiling with your elbow bent.

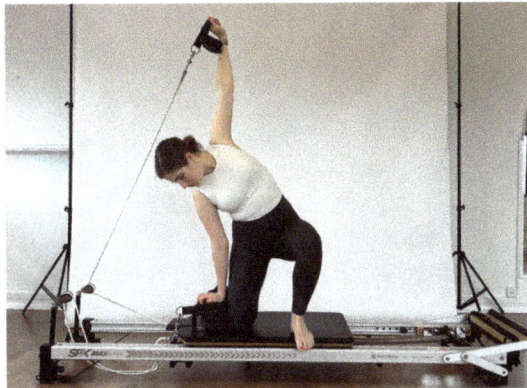

B
EXHALE

1. Pull the strap straightening your elbow and your hand reaches up to the ceiling.

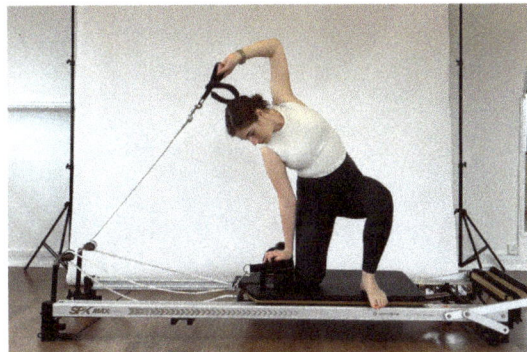

C
INHALE

1. Return to position **A**.
2. Repeat on the other side.

VARIATION

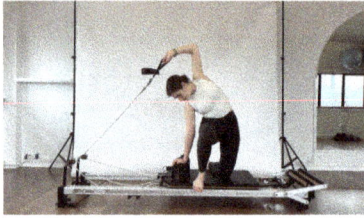

1. Swap your legs **(A)**

PROGRESSION

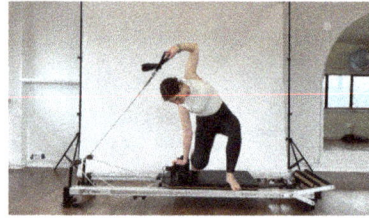

1. Lift your back knee off the carriage **(A)**

ANTI-GRAVITY I

Strength: Chest, shoulder, abs, tricep, quads

Level: Intermediate   **Repetition:** 8-10   **Springs:** Light to medium

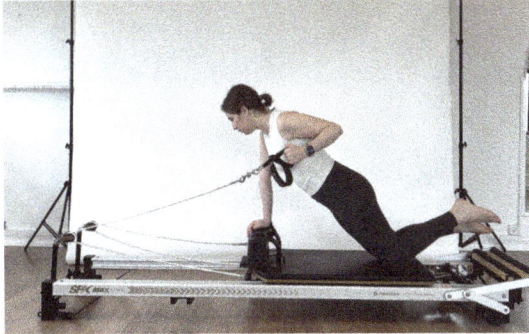

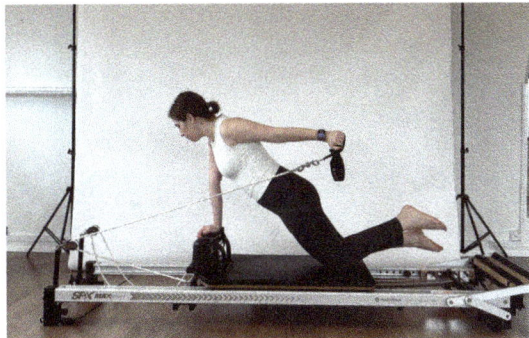

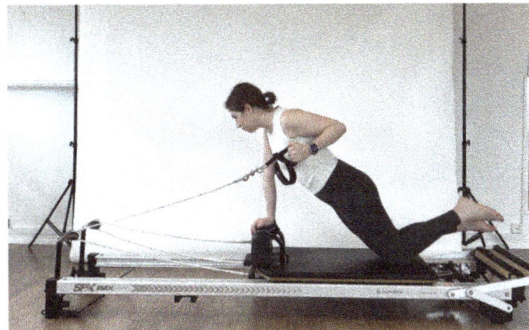

A
START

1. Face the riser end and bring your body into a high kneeling plank position. Place one hand on the shoulder rest.
2. Hold onto the strap bringing your upper arm slightly behind you and the arm in line with the sides of your ribs. Your elbow is bent.

B
EXHALE

1. Extend your arms behind you.

C
INHALE

1. Return to position **A**.
2. Repeat on the other side.

VARIATION

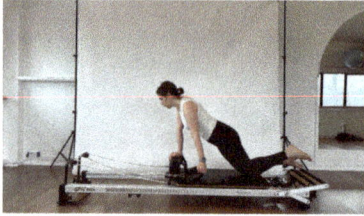

1. Pull the strap behind you keeping your elbow straight **(A)**

PROGRESSION 1

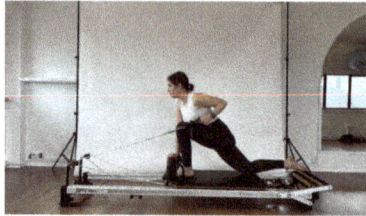

1. Bring the opposite leg forward placing it on top of the headrest. The other knee is behind your hip on the carriage. Elbow is bent to start **(A)**

PROGRESSION 2

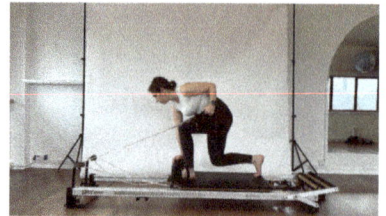

1. Lift the back knee off. The knee is directly below your hip. Elbow is bent to start **(A)**

PROGRESSION 3

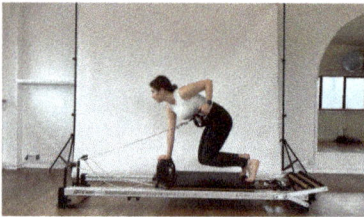

1. Lift both knees off. Toes are tucked and knees directly below your hips **(A)**

ANTI-GRAVITY II

Strength: Chest, shoulder, arms, abs, tricep, quads

Level: Intermediate   **Repetition:** 8-10   **Springs:** Light to medium

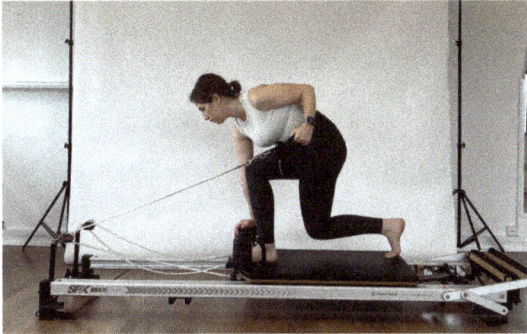

A
START

1. Kneel on the carriage with one foot on the headrest and the other knee lifted off the carriage directly below the hip.
2. Place the one hand on top of the shoulder rest and the other hand hold the strap with the elbow bent and directly behind the shoulder.

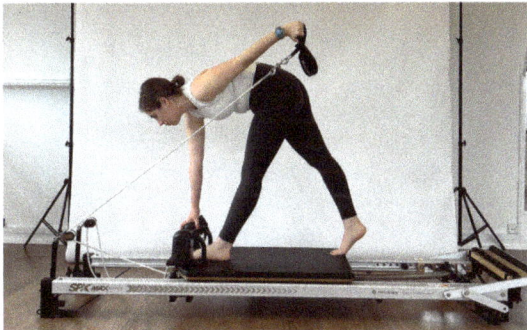

B
EXHALE

1. Extend your elbow bringing your hand to the wall behind you at the same time as you extend both knees. Continue holding onto the shoulder rest.

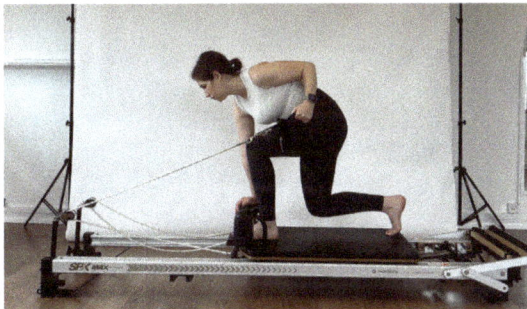

C
INHALE

1. Return to position **A**
2. Repeat on the other side

VARIATION

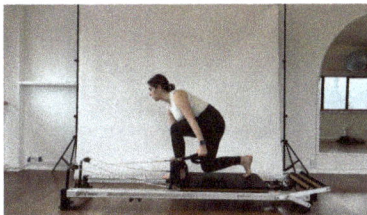

1. Extend your elbow and pull the straight arm backward **(A)**

ANTI-GRAVITY III

Strength: Chest, shoulder,arms, abs, tricep, quads

Level: Intermediate   **Repetition:** 8-10   **Springs:**Light to medium

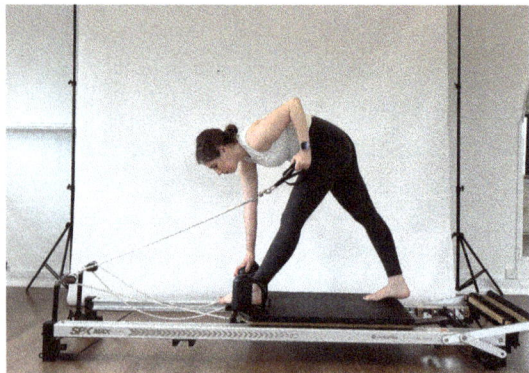

A
START

1. Stand on the carriage with one foot on the headrest and the other leg extended behind with your toes on the edge of the carriage.
2. Place the one hand on top of the shoulder rest and the other hand hold the strap with the elbow bent and directly behind the shoulder.

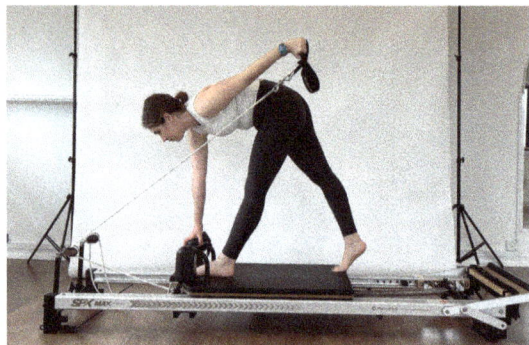

B
EXHALE

1. Extend your elbow pulling the strap.

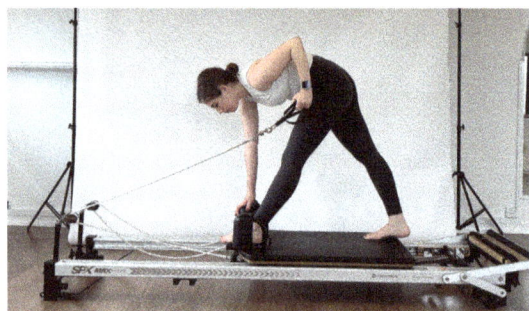

C
INHALE

1. Return to position **A**.
2. Repeat on the other side.

VARIATION

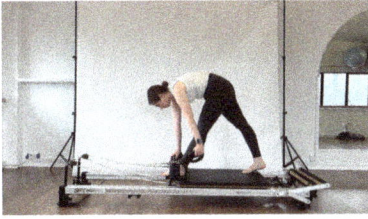

1. Pull a straight arm backward **(A)**

PROGRESSION 1

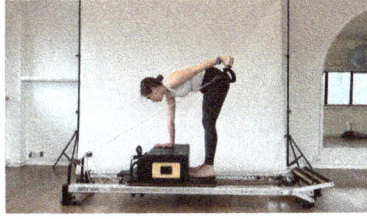

1. Place the reformer box in the short box position. Stand on top of the carriage facing the risers. Bend both knees, hip hinge and place one hand on the box the other pulls the arm backward holding the strap **(B)**

PROGRESSION 2

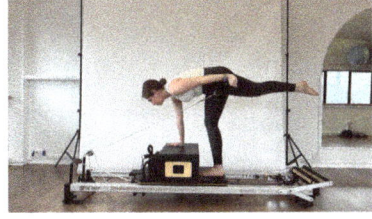

1. Extend one leg back with the same position as the previous progression **(B)**

PETER PAN I

Strength: Shoulder, bicep, oblique, glutes, quads

Level: Intermediate   **Repetition:** 8-10   **Springs:** Light to medium

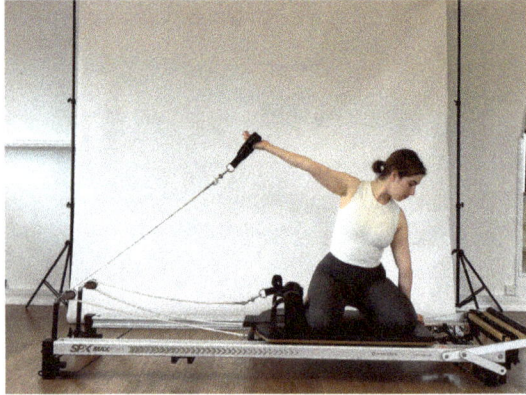

A

START

1. Sit sideways on the carriage with both legs bent and your feet pointing backward. Your hip is on the carriage toward the footbar end.
2. Place the footbar end hand on the carriage and hold onto the strap with your other hand.
3. Extend your elbow bringing your strap hand in line with the shoulder to the side of your body.

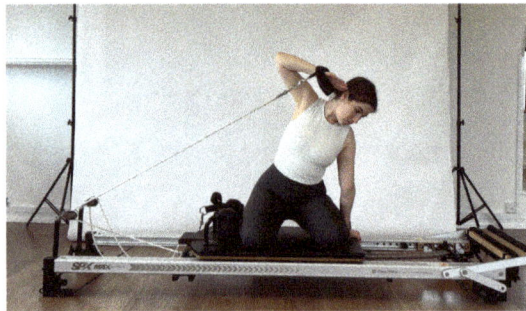

B

INHALE

1. Bend your elbow bringing your hand toward your head.

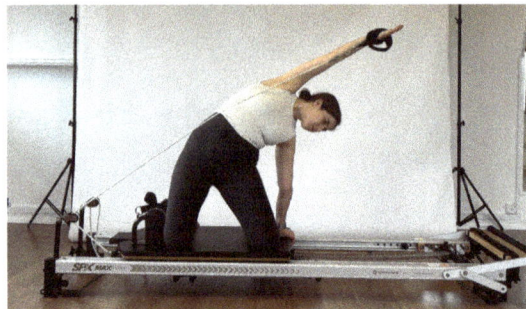

C

EXHALE

1. Bend sideways toward the footbar extending your arm. Continue the curve created by the side bend.

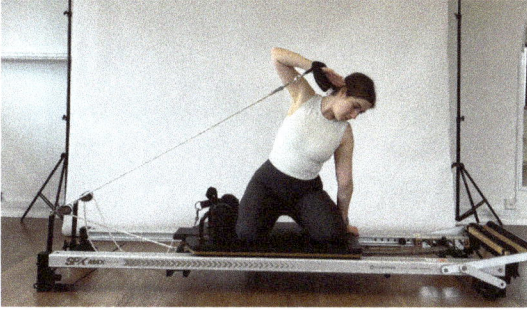

D

INHALE

1. Return to position **B**.

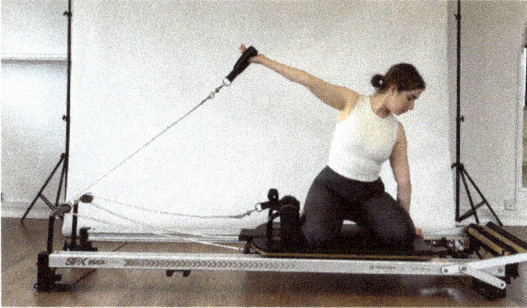

E

EXHALE

1. Return to position **A**.
2. Repeat on the other side.

PETER PAN II

Strength: Shoulder, bicep, oblique, glutes, hamstrings

Level: Intermediate   **Repetition:** 8-10   **Springs:** Light to medium

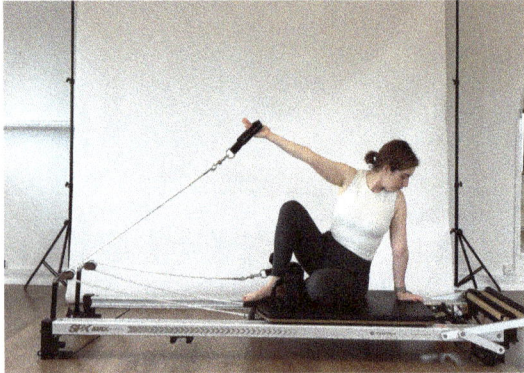

A
START

1. Sit sideways on the carriage. Place one foot on the headrest and the other leg is bent with your shin against the shoulder rests.
2. Hold onto the strap with your arm extended out in line with your shoulder with the hand closest to the risers. The other hand rests on the carriage.

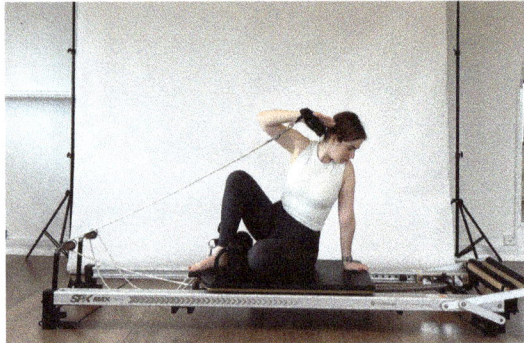

B
INHALE

1. Bend your elbow bringing your fingers toward your ears.

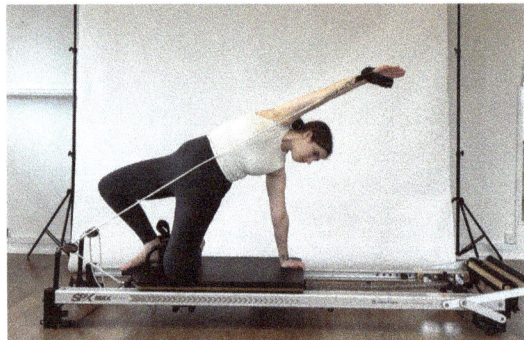

C
EXHALE

1. Lift your hips, extend arm overhead and create a side bend with your spine.

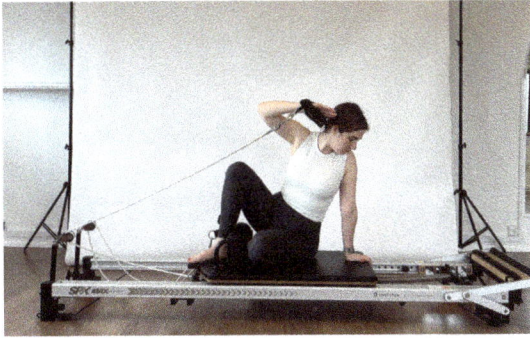

D

INHALE

1. Return to position **B**

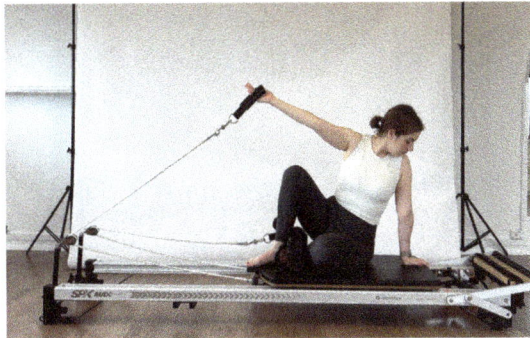

E

EXHALE

1. Return to position **A**.
2. Repeat on the other side.

PETER PAN III

Strength: Shoulder, biceps, obliques, glutes, hamstrings

Level: Intermediate   **Repetition:** 8-10   **Springs:** Light to medium

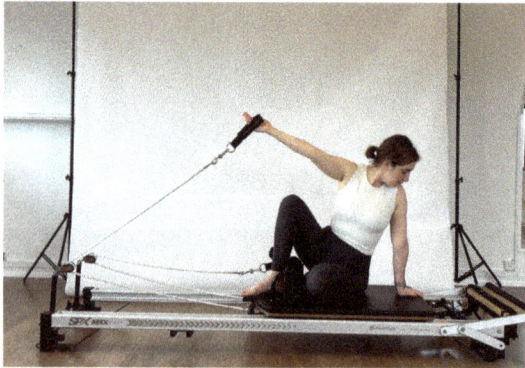

A
START

1. Sit sideways on the carriage. Place one foot on the headrest and the other leg is bent with your shin against the shoulder rests.
2. Hold onto the strap with your arm extended out in line with your shoulder with the hand closest to the risers. The other hand rests on the carriage.

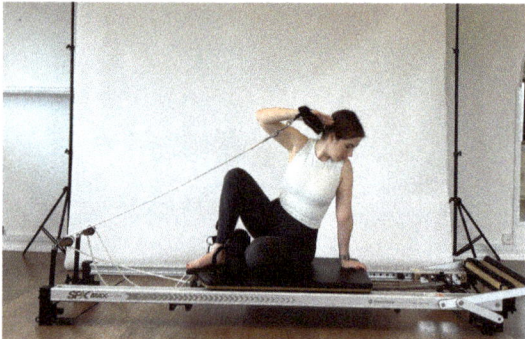

B
INHALE

1. Bend your elbow bringing your fingers toward your ears.

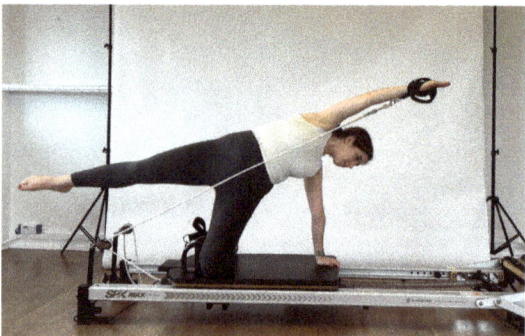

C
EXHALE

1. Bend sideways toward the footbar extending your arm. Continue the curve created by the side bend.
2. Extend your headrest leg out to the side as high as your hip.

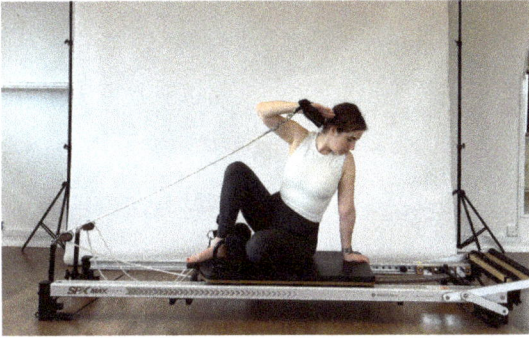

D

INHALE

1. Return to position **B**.

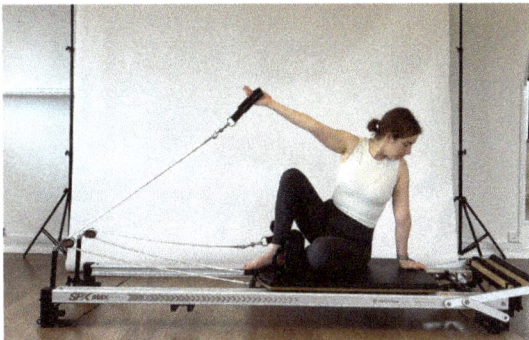

E

EXHALE

1. Returnto position **A**.
2. Repeat on the other side.

PETER PAN IV

Strength: Shoulder, biceps, obliques, quads

Level: Intermediate   **Repetition:** 8-10   **Springs:** light to medium

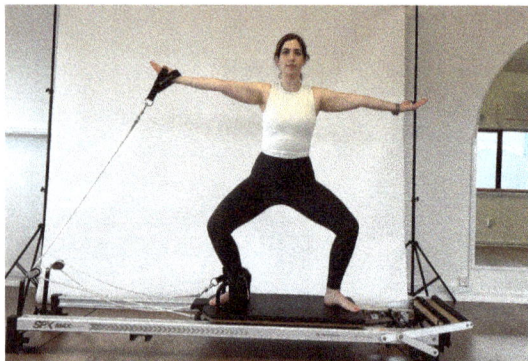

A
START

1. Stand sideways on the carriage. The legs are turned out and knees bent. Hold onto one strap with the hand closest to the risers.
2. Extend both arms out to the side at shoulder level.

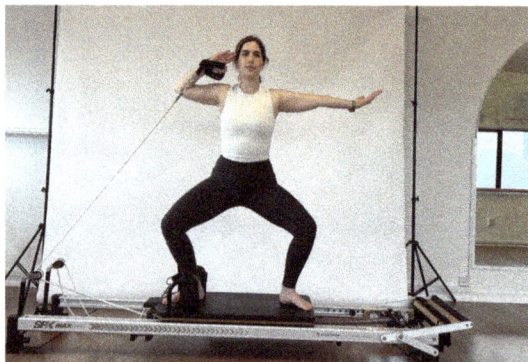

B
INHALE

1. Bend the strap arm elbow bringing the hand toward your ear.

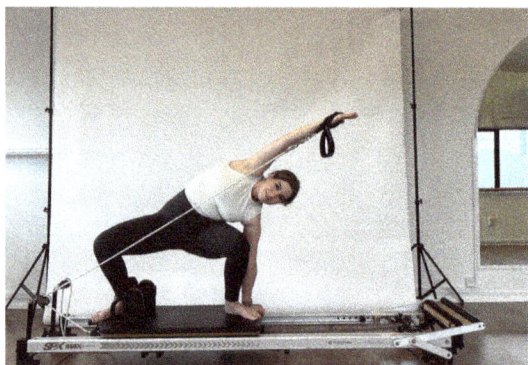

C
EXHALE

1. Bend sideways toward the footbar extending the arm overhead.

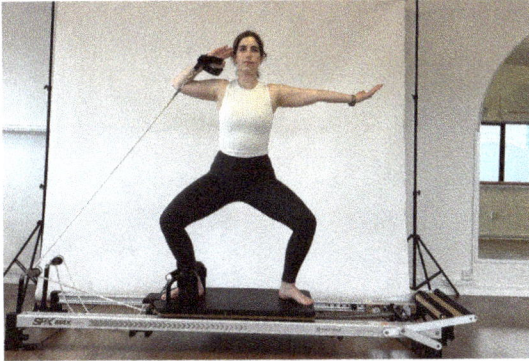

D

INHALE

1. Return to position B

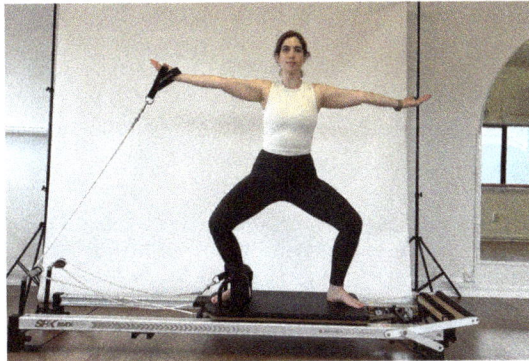

E

EXHALE

1. Return to position **A**.
2. Repeat on the other side.

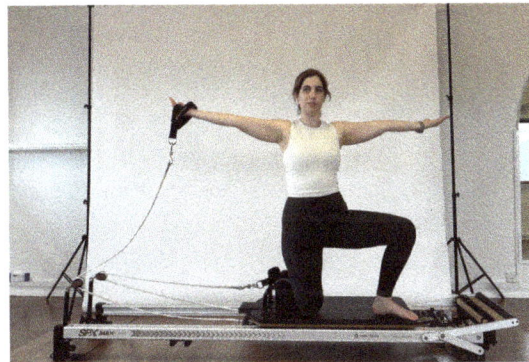

MODIFICATION

1. Kneel on the carriage with the knee closest to the shoulder rests on the carriage and the other leg in the open position.

BAMBOO SWAY I

Strength: Shoulder, arms, obliques

Level: Intermediate   **Repetition:** 8-10   **Springs:** Light to medium

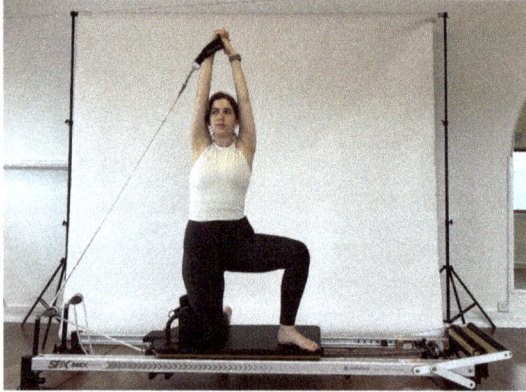

A
START

1. Kneel sideways on the carriage in an open kneel position. One leg is pressing against the shoulder rests with the knee under the hip. The other leg is turned out. The other foot is placed on the front corner of the carriage slightly turned out.
2. Both hands hold onto the strap with the hands clasped overhead.

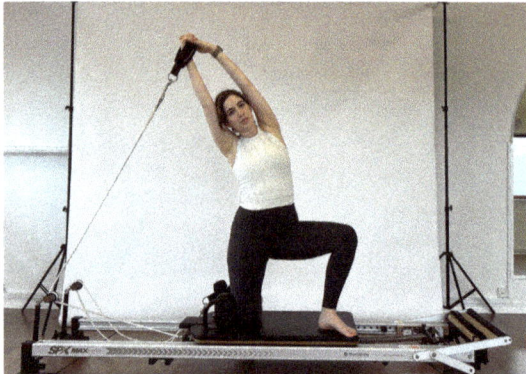

B
INHALE

1. Bend sideways toward the risers.

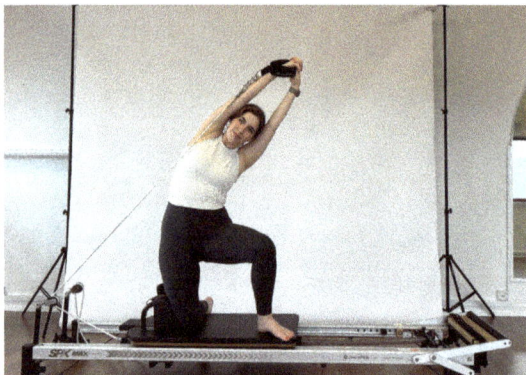

C
EXHALE

1. Bend over toward the footbar.

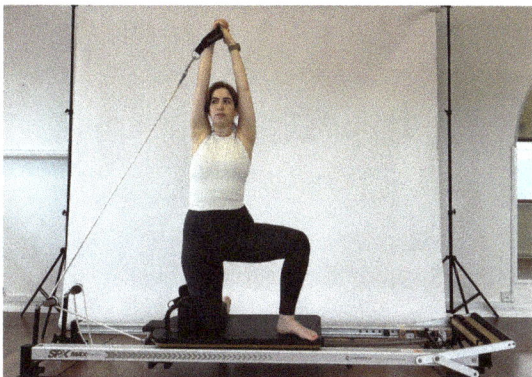

D
INHALE

1. Return to position **B**.
2. Repeat on the other side.

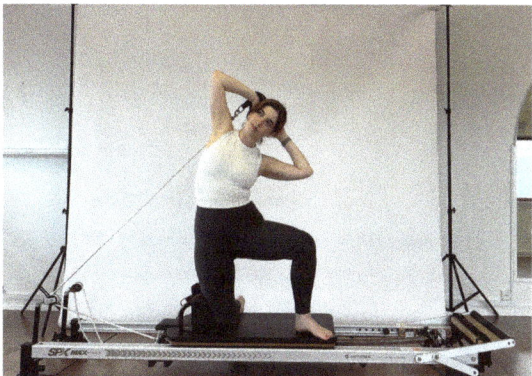

MODIFICATION

1. Place your hands behind your head.

BAMBOO SWAY II

Strength: Shoulder, arms, obliques

Level: Intermediate   **Repetition:** 8-10   **Springs:** Light to medium

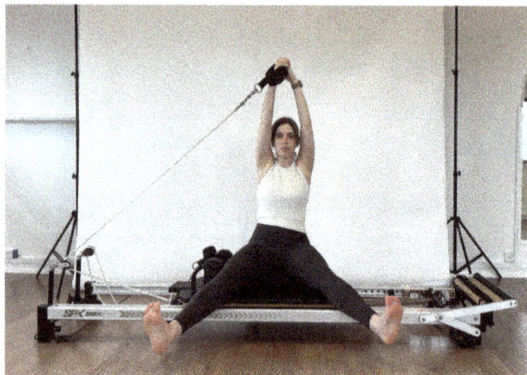

A
START

1. Sitting sideways on the carriage in a straddle position.
2. Extend both arms overhead holding one strap

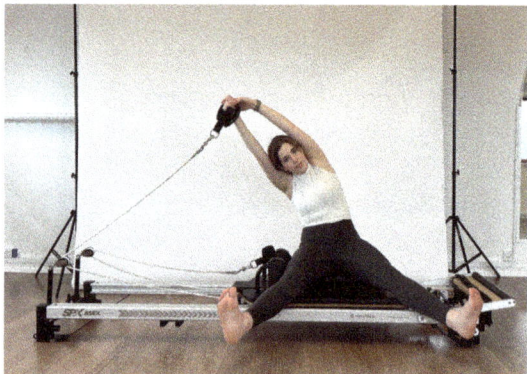

B
EXHALE

1. Bend sideways toward the risers.

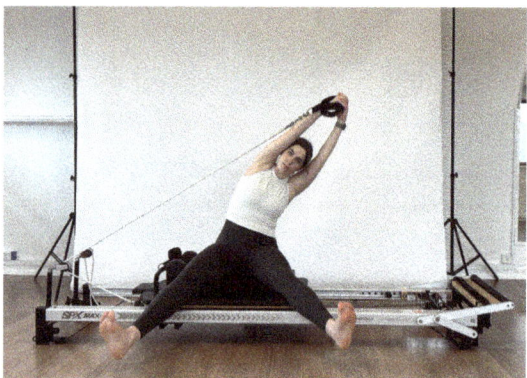

C
INHALE

1. Bend sideways toward the footbar.

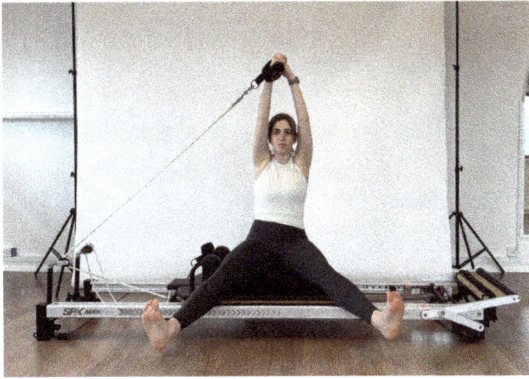

D
EXHALE

1. Return to position **A**.
2. Repeat on the other side.

BAMBOO SWING

Strength: Shoulders, arms, obliques

Level: Intermediate **Repetition:** 8-10 **Springs:** Light to medium

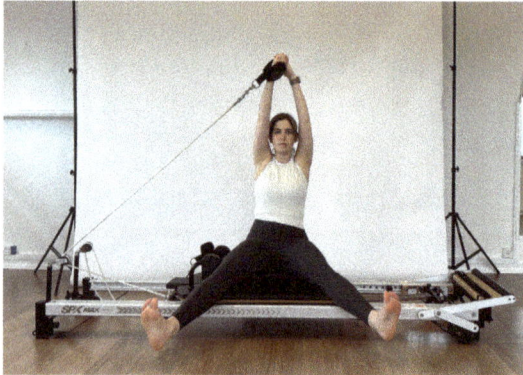

A
START

1. Sitting sideways on the carriage in a straddle position.
2. Extend both arms overhead holding one strap.

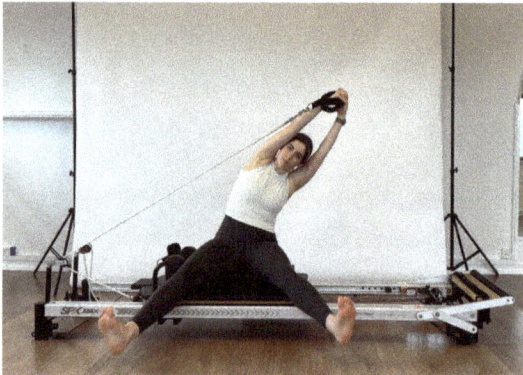

B
EXHALE

1. Bend towards the footbar

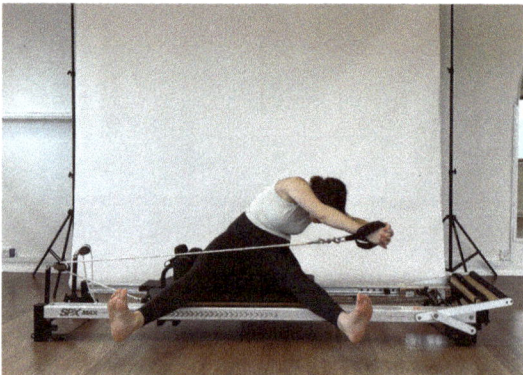

C
INHALE

1. Twist your spine. Your breastbone faces your leg on the same side as the side bend.

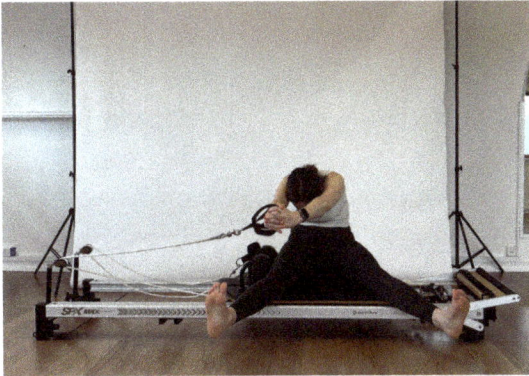

D

EXHALE

1. Move your body over to the opposite leg maintaining a flexed spine.

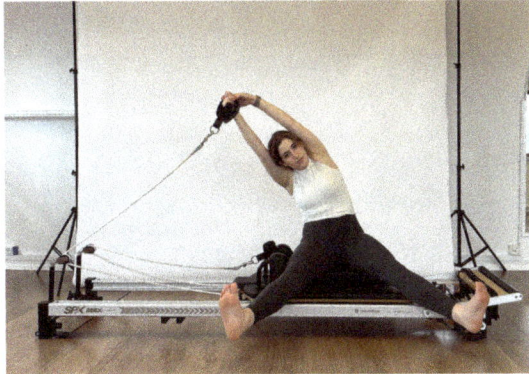

E

INHALE

1. Lift your trunk into a side bend to the other side. Your chest faces to the front.

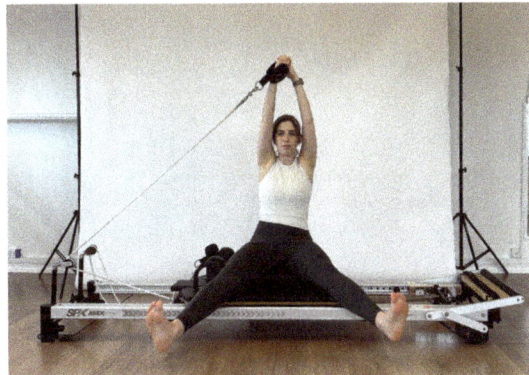

F

INHALE

1. Return to position **A**.
2. Repeat on the other side.

FLIP SIDE I

Strength: Shoulder, bicep, quads, glutes

Level: Intermediate   **Repetition:** 8-10   **Springs:** light to medium

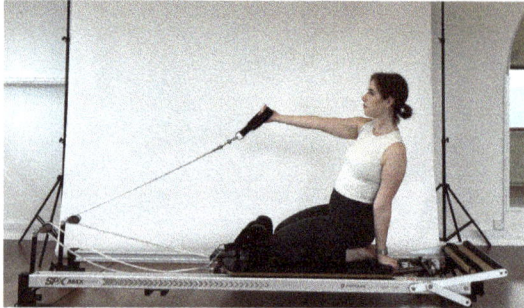

A
START

1. Japanese kneeling position on the carriage facing the risers.
2. Place one hand slightly behind you on the corner of the carriage. The other hand holds the strap with the elbow extended out in line with your shoulder.

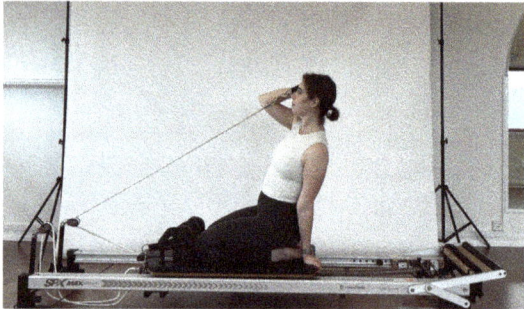

B
INHALE

1. Bend your elbow bringing your strap hand closer to your head.

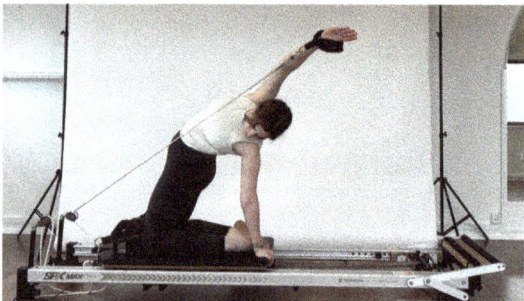

C
EXHALE

1. Simultaneously push your hips up as you twist toward your carriage hand and extend your arm overhead.

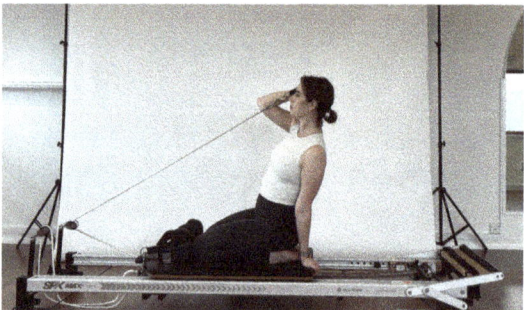

D
INHALE

1. Return to position **B**.

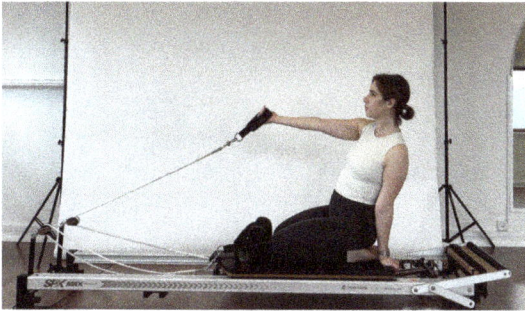

E
EXHALE

1. Return to position **A**.
2. Repeat on the other side.

PROGRESSION

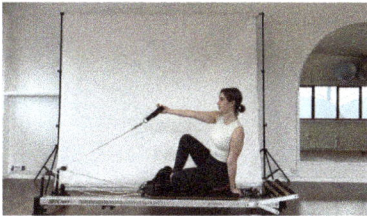

1. One leg bend pointing to the ceiling while you are sitting on top of your other foot. **(A)**

FLIP SIDE II

Strength: Back, shoulders, biceps, quads, glutes, hamstrings

Level: Intermediate   **Repetition:** 8-10   **Springs:** Light to medium

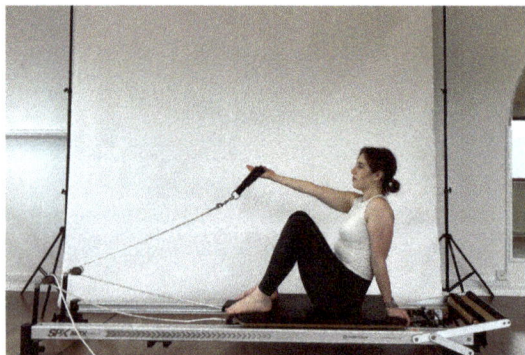

A
START

1. Sit on the carriage facing the risers.
2. Both knees are bent and the feet are on the corners.
3. Place one hand on the corner of the carriage behind you. The other hand holds the strap with your elbow extended and hand as high as the shoulder.

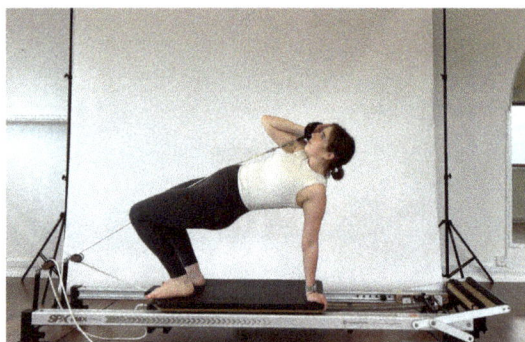

B
EXHALE

1. Press heels and rear hand down to lift your hips up. Pull the strap towards your shoulder, bending your elbow.

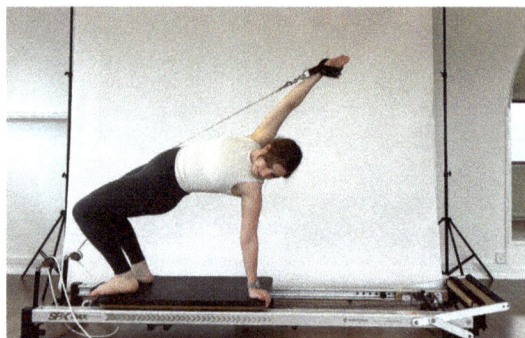

C
INHALE

1. Twist your spine toward the supporting arm as you extend your arm overhead.

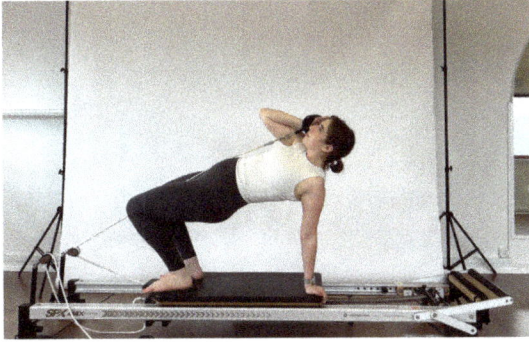

D
EXHALE

1. Return to position **B**.

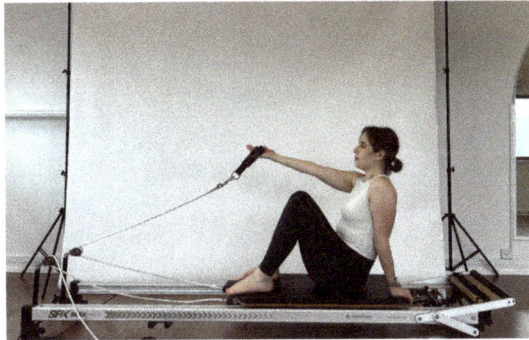

E
INHALE

1. Return to position **A**.
2. Repeat on the other side.

UNTOLD
PART VI

SWORDFISH I

Strength: Chest, shoulders, arms, abs

Level: Intermediate   **Repetition:** 8-10   **Springs:** Medium

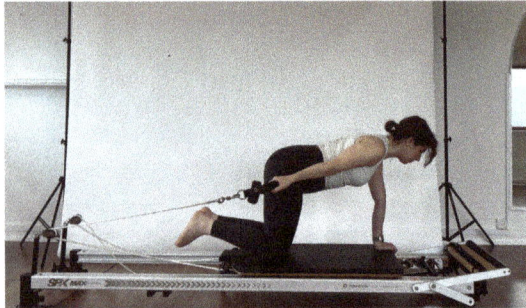

A
START

1. Neutral, four point kneeling facing the footbar.
2. Hold onto one of the straps with the arm lined up next to your body.

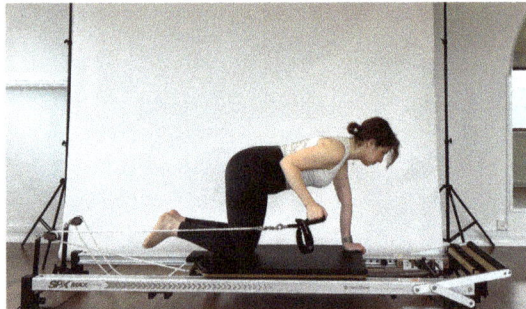

B
EXHALE

1. Bend your elbow keeping your upper arm where it is.

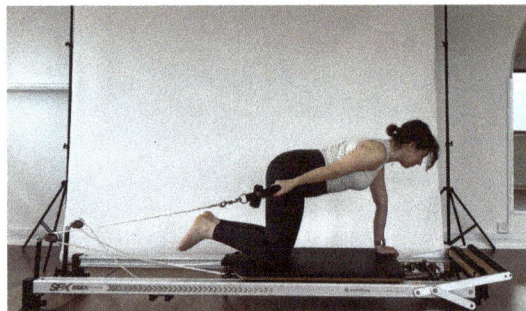

C
INHALE

1. Straighten your elbow.
2. Repeat on the other side.

PROGRESSION 1

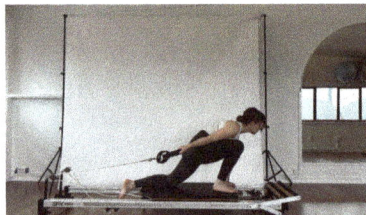

1. Bring one foot forward. Place the foot on the carriage with the knee bent at 90 degrees. Tuck the toes of the leg behind. **(B)**

PROGRESSION 2

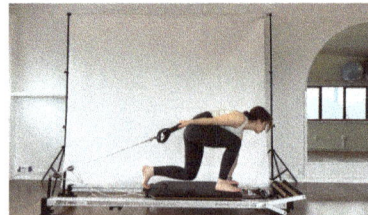

1. Tuck the toes of the back foot and lift the knee off slightly **(A)**

SWORDFISH II

Strength: Chest, shoulders, arms, abs

Level: Intermediate +   **Repetition:** 8-10   **Springs:** Medium

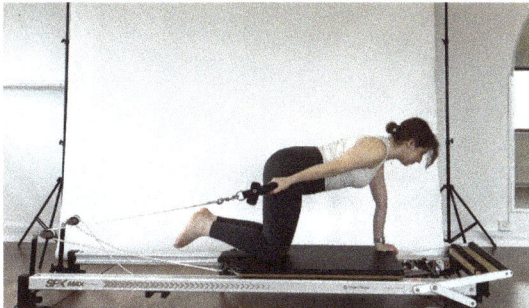

A
START

1. Neutral, four point kneeling facing the footbar.
2. Hold onto one of the straps with the arm lined up next to your body.

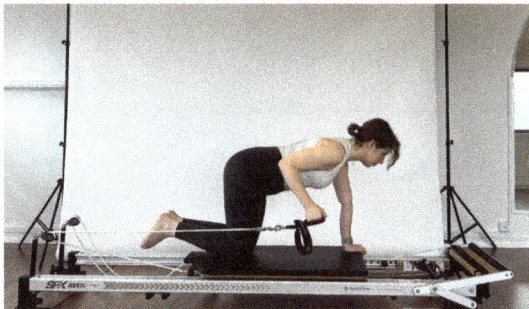

B
EXHALE

1. Bend your elbow keeping your upper arm where it is.

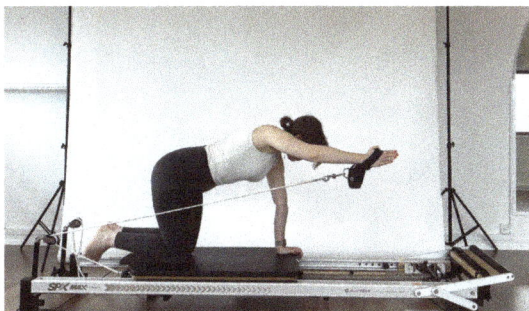

C
INHALE

1. Extend the arm forward toward the wall in front of you.

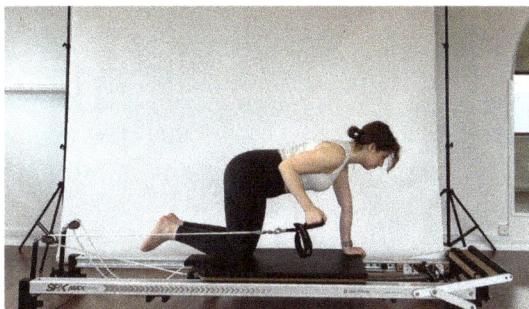

D
EXHALE

1. Bend the elbow bringing the upper arm next to your ribs

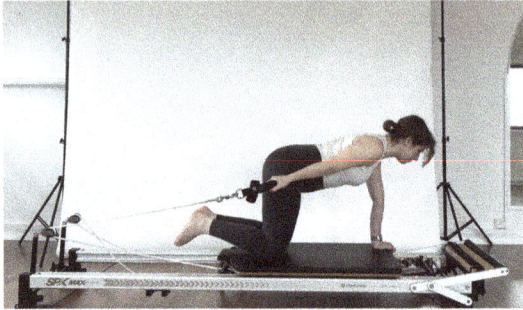

E

INHALE

1. Straighten the elbow extending the hand behind you.
2. Repeat on the other side.

PROGRESSION 1

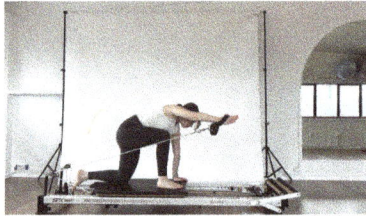

1. Bring one foot forward. Place the foot on the carriage with the knee bent at 90 degrees. Tuck the toes of the leg behind. **(C)**

PROGRESSION 2

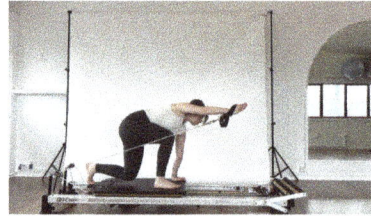

1. Tuck the toes of the back foot and lift the knee off slightly. **(C)**

SWORDFISH III

Strength: Chest, shoulders, arms, obliques

Level: Intermediate   **Repetition:** 8-10   **Springs:** Medium

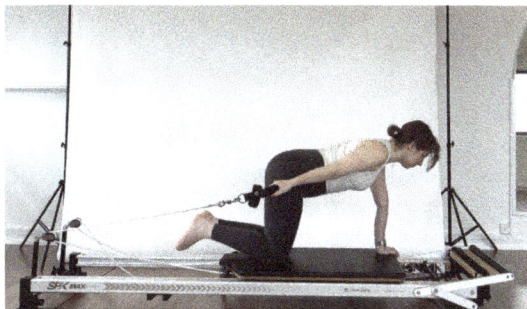

A
START

1. Neutral, four point kneeling facing the footbar.
2. Hold onto one of the straps with the arm lined up next to your body.

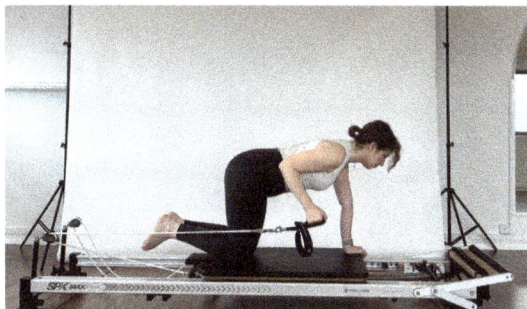

B
EXHALE

1. Bend the elbow and bring the hand below the shoulder

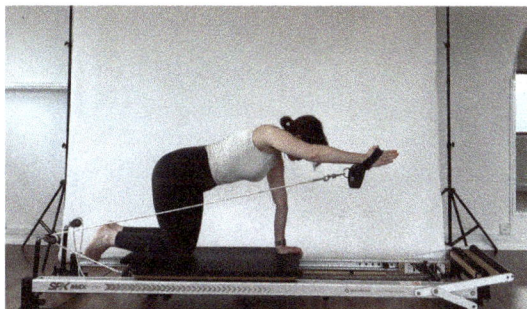

C
INHALE

1. Extend the arm forward toward the wall in front of you.

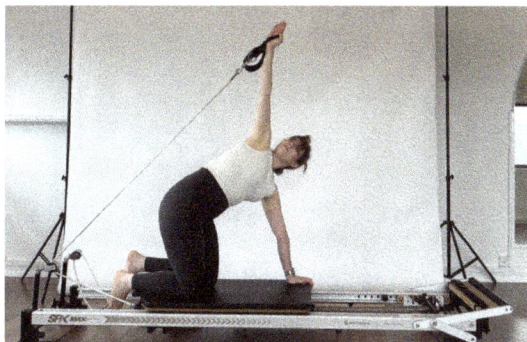

D
EXHALE

1. Rotate your spine, reaching your hand up to the ceiling.

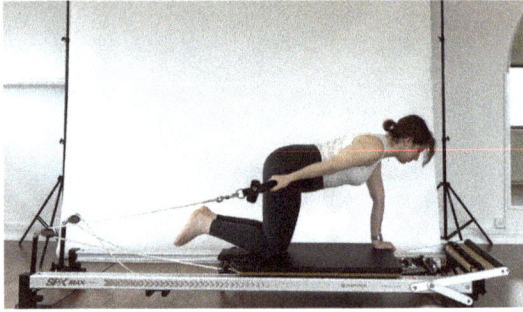

E

INHALE

1. Circle your arm back to position **A**.
2. Repeat on the other side.

PROGRESSION 1

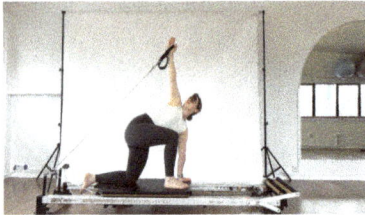

1. Bring one foot forward. Place the foot on the carriage with the knee bent at 90 degrees. Tuck the toes of the leg behind. **(D)**

PROGRESSION 2

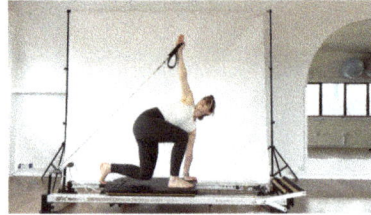

1. Tuck the toes of the back foot and lift the knee off slightly. **(D)**

SWORDFISH IV

Strength: Chest, shoulders, arms, obliques, glutes, hamstrings

Level: Intermediate   **Repetition:** 8-10   **Springs:** Medium

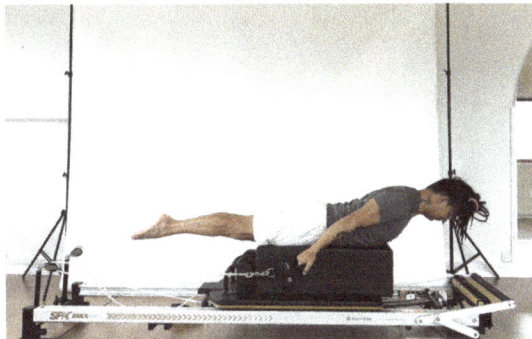

A

START

1. Lie on your belly on the box facing the footbar.
2. Place one hand on the carriage. The other hand holds the strap.
3. Legs are extended and together.

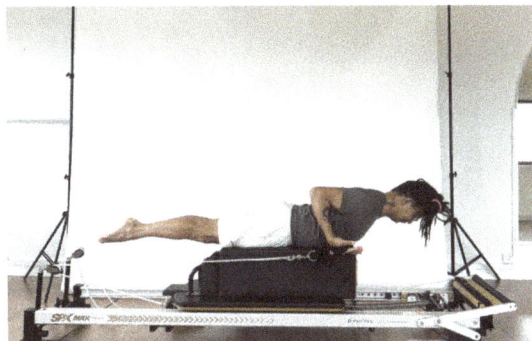

B

EXHALE

1. Bend the elbow and bring the hand below the shoulder.

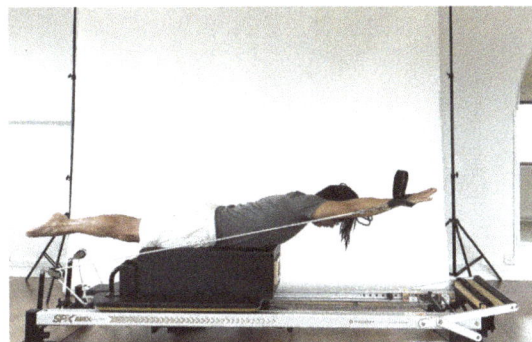

C

INHALE

1. Extend the arm forward toward the wall in front of you.

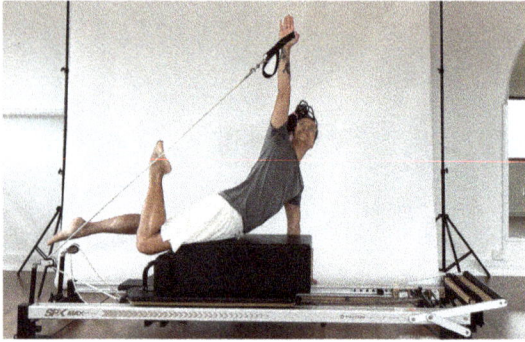

D
EXHALE

1. Rotate your spine, reaching your hand toward the ceiling as you press into your carriage hand. Your torso will lift off the box.
2. Bend the knee of the same leg as the strap hand.

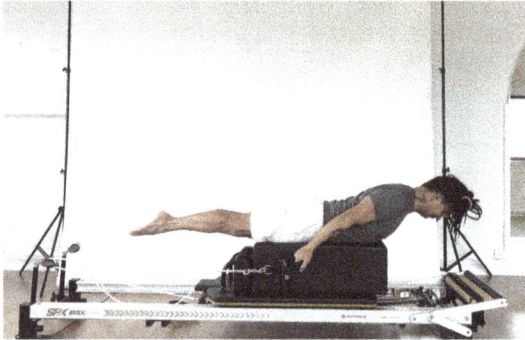

E
INHALE

1. Circle back to position **A**.
2. Repeat on the other side.

BAT WING I

Strength: Chest, shoulders, arms, obliques

Level: Intermediate   **Repetition:** 8-10   **Springs:** Light to medium

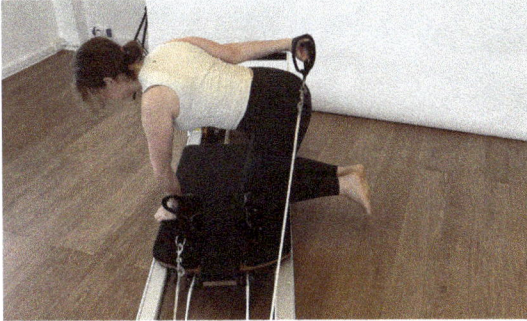

A
START

1. Four point kneeling sideways across the carriage
2. The footbar hand holds the rear strap above the tailbone.

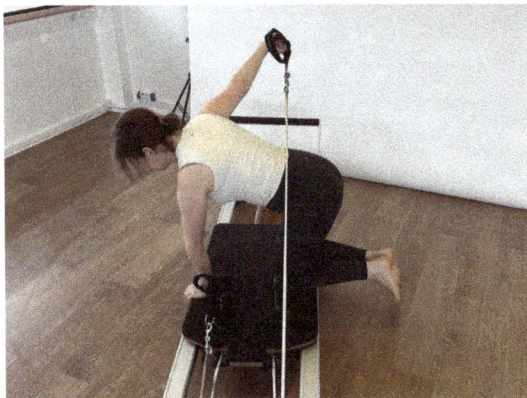

B
EXHALE

1. Open the strap arm towards the footbar staying at shoulder height.

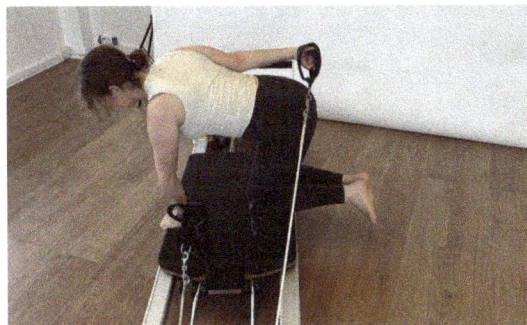

C
INHALE

1. Return to position **A**.
2. Repeat on the other side.

BAT WING II

Strength: Chest, shoulders, arms, obliques

Level: Intermediate   **Repetition:** 8-10   **Springs:** Light to medium

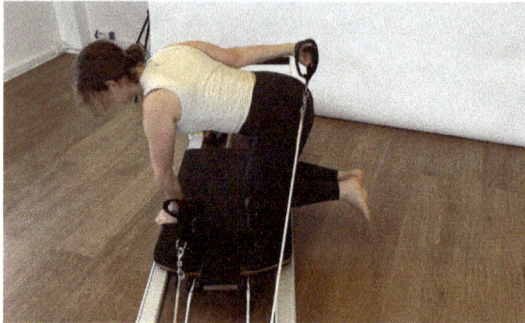

A
START

1. Four point kneeling sideways across the carriage
2. The footbar hand holds the rear strap above the tailbone.

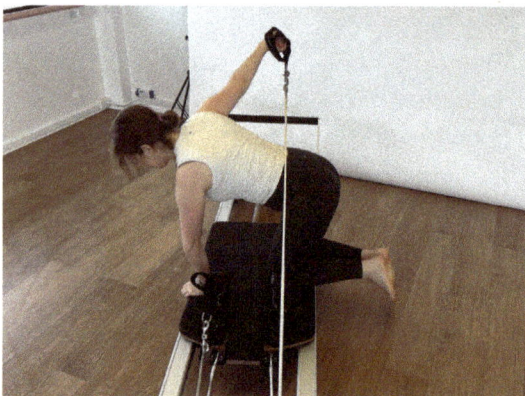

B
EXHALE

1. Open the strap arm towards the footbar staying at shoulder height.

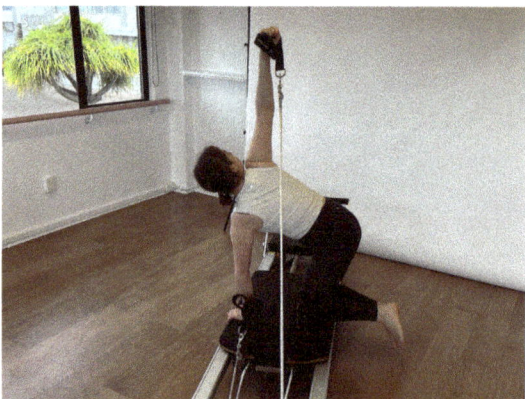

C
INHALE

1. Rotate your trunk so your arm reaches up to the ceiling.

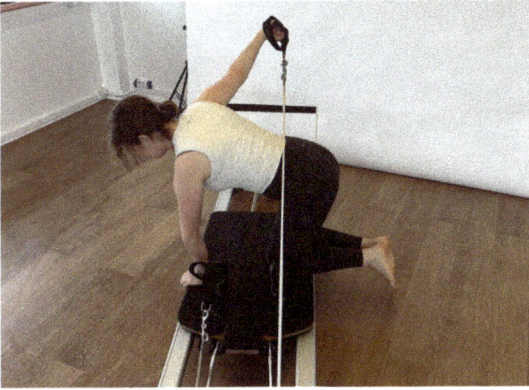

D

EXHALE

1. Return to position **B**.

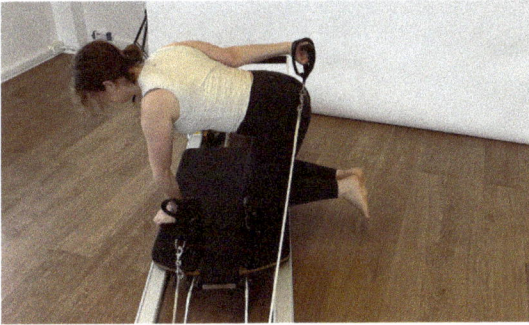

E

INHALE

1. Return to position **A**.
2. Repeat on the other side.

TWISTER I

Strength: Shoulders, arms, obliques

Level: Intermediate   **Repetition:** 8-10   **Springs:** Light to medium

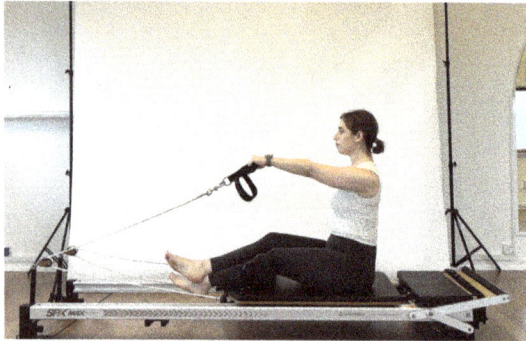

A
START

1. Sitting in neutral spine, facing the risers.
2. Hold onto one strap. Your other hand holds the hip.
3. Cross your ankles

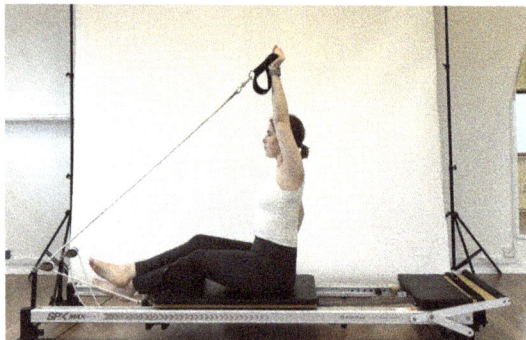

B
EXHALE

1. Lift the arm up toward the ceiling.

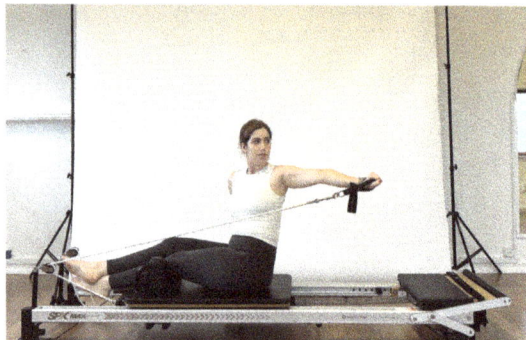

C
INHALE

1. Rotate your ribs, lowering the arm towards the footbar and twisting your ribs toward the same side.
2. Keep your shoulders down from the entire rotation.

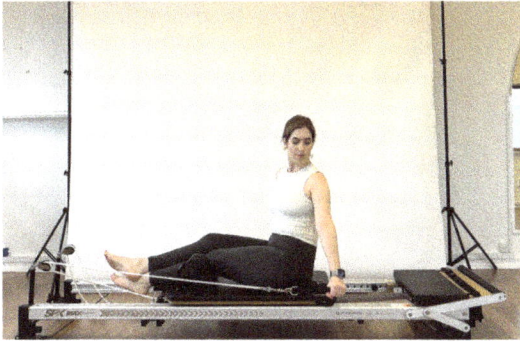

D

EXHALE

1. Lower the arm next to your body and rotate your ribs to face the risers.

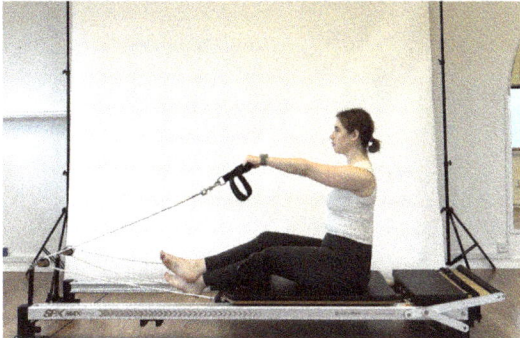

E

INHALE

1. Return to position **A**.
2. Repeat on the other side.

TWISTER II

Strength: Shoulders, arms, obliques, triceps

Level: Intermediate   **Repetition:** 8-10   **Springs:** Medium

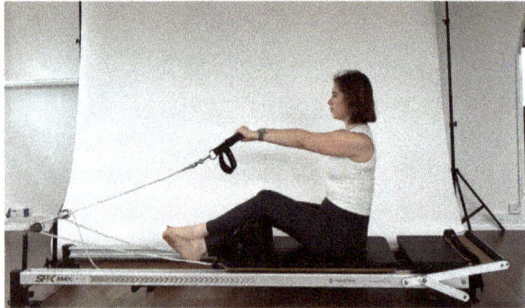

A
START

1. Sit upright in neutral spine facing the risers.
2. Bring both hands forward and lift them to shoulder height. One hand holds the strap.
3. Cross your ankles.

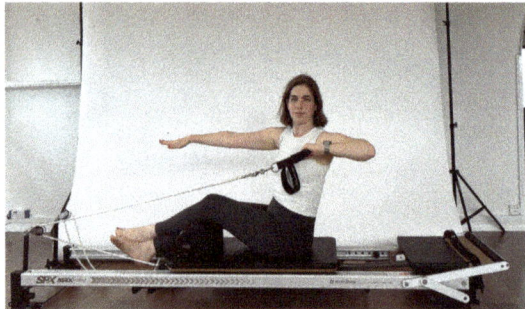

B
EXHALE

1. Rotate your ribs while bending your elbow in line with your shoulder.

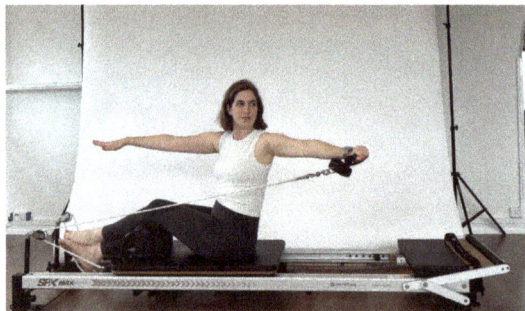

C
INHALE

1. Straighten your elbow, extending your hand toward the wall behind you.

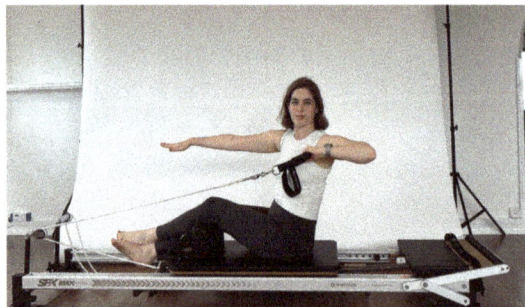

D
EXHALE

1. Bend your elbow back to position **B**.

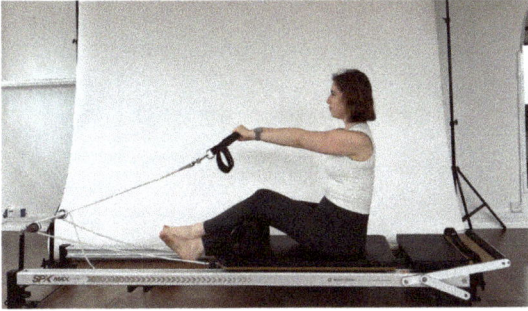

E.

INHALE

1. Return to position **A**.
2. Repeat on the other side.

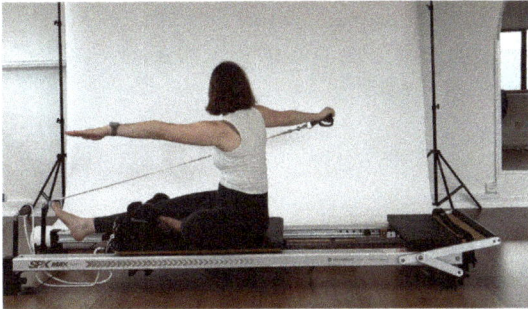

MODIFICATION

1. Place the opposite foot next to the knee of the straight leg. Rotate the knee toward the carriage (frog leg) **C.**

PROGRESSION

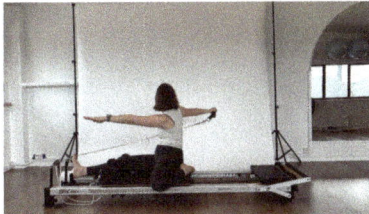

1. Tuck the opposite foot behind your bottom. **(C)**

TWISTER III

Strength: Shoulders, arms, obliques, triceps

Level: Intermediate   **Repetition:** 8-10   **Springs**: Medium

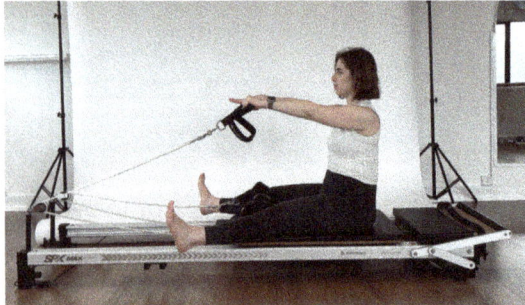

A
START

1. Sit upright in neutral spine facing the risers.
2. Bring both hands forward and lift them to shoulder height. One hand holds the strap.
3. Extend both legs in front of you as wide as the carriage. Your legs are on the outside of the shoulder rests.

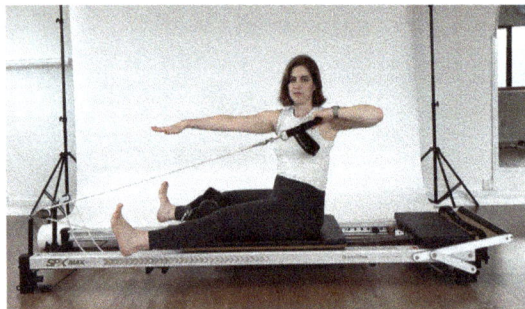

B
EXHALE

1. Rotate your ribs and bend your elbow keeping the arm at shoulder height.

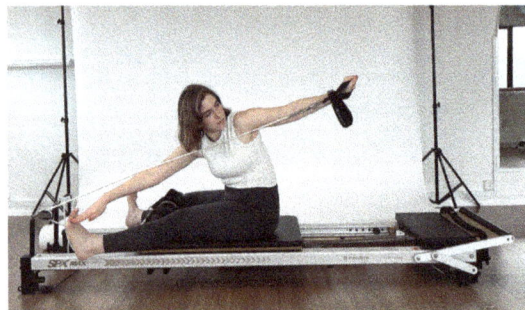

C
INHALE

1. Reach your free hand across to the opposite foot like the mat exercise Saw.
2. Extend your elbow reaching your strap arm to the wall behind you as you lean forward.

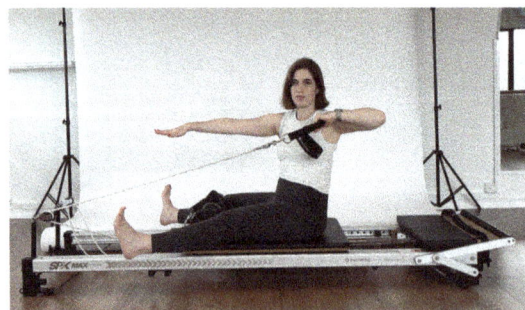

D
EXHALE

1. Return to position **B**.

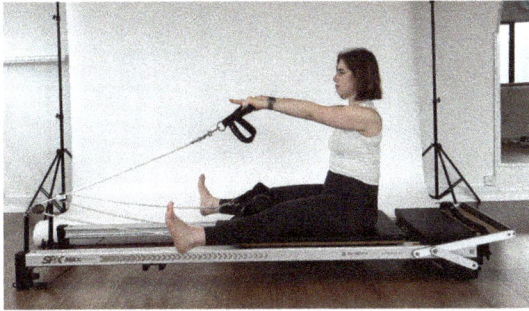

E
INHALE

1. Return to position **A**.
2. Repeat on the other side.

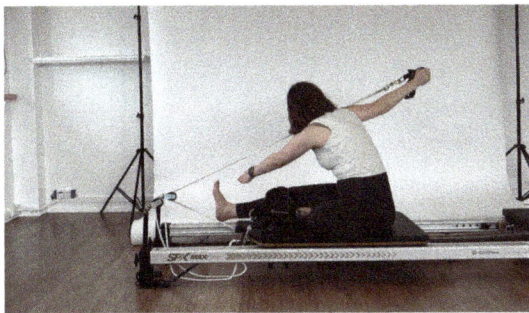

MODIFICATION

1. Place the opposite foot next to the knee of the straight leg. Rotate the knee toward the carriage (frog leg) **C**

PROGRESSION

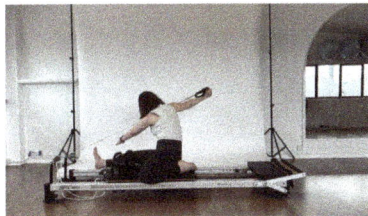

1. Tuck the opposite foot behind your bottom.**(C)**

TWISTER IV

Strength: Shoulders, arms, obliques, quads

Level: Intermediate   **Repetition:** 8-10   **Springs:** Medium

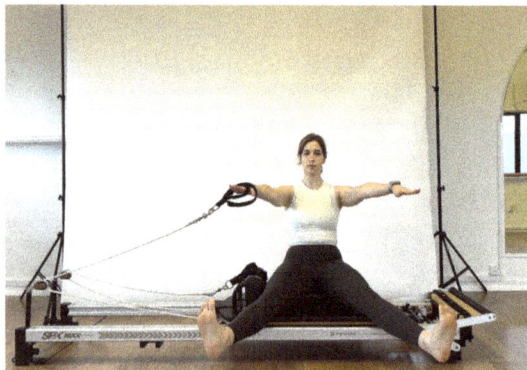

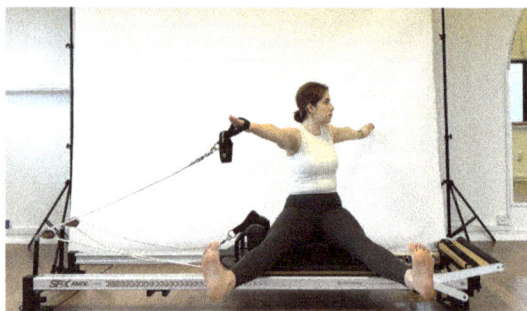

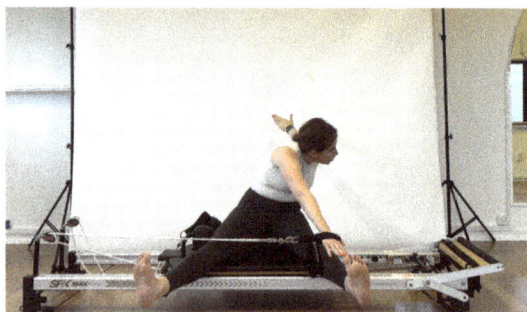

A

START

1. Neutral spine, sitting sideways on the carriage. Place your legs in a straddle position with your feet toward the corners of the carriage. Flex your feet. Remove the shoulder pads if you can.
2. Both arms align over your legs at shoulder height. The arm closest to the risers holds the strap.

B

EXHALE

1. Rotate your spine toward the footbar.
2. Reach back with your free arm.

C

INHALE

1. Lean forward as you reach to the outside of your opposite foot with your strap arm.

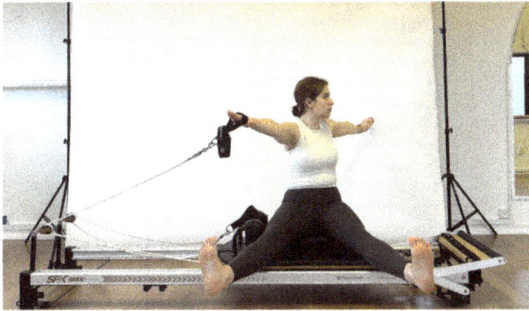

D

EXHALE

1. Return to position **B**.

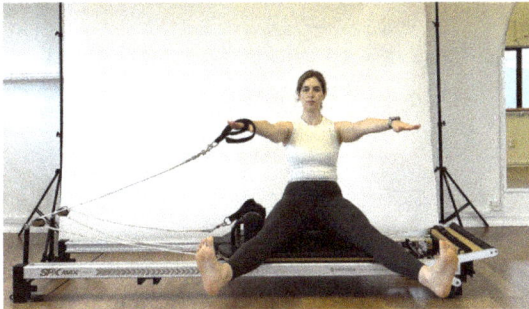

E

INHALE

1. Return to position **A**.
2. Repeat on the other side.

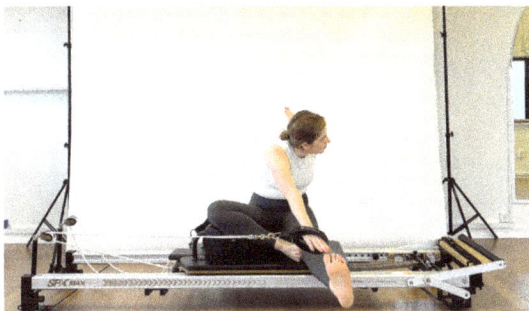

MODIFICATION

1. Turn the shoulder rest leg outward into a frog position. Bring the other leg forward **C.**

CORK BORER PREP

Strength: Shoulders, arms, obliques

Level: Intermediate   **Repetition:** 8-10   **Springs:** Light to medium

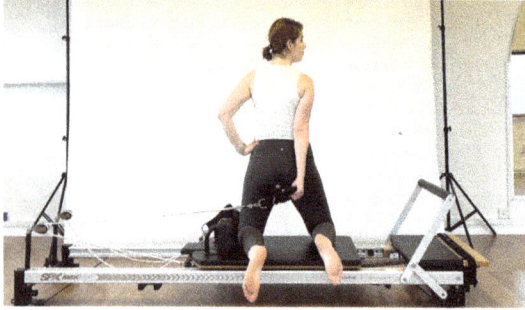

A
START

1. High kneeling facing sideways on the carriage with your legs shoulder width apart.
2. The footbar hand holds the back strap slightly behind the body.

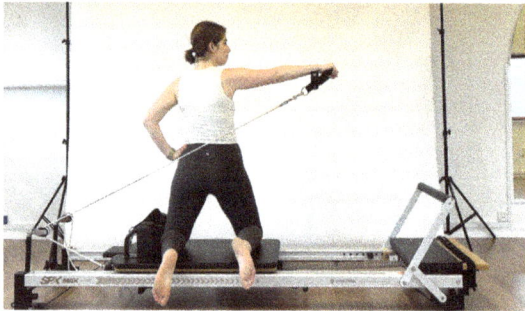

B
EXHALE

1. Lift your arm sideways to shoulder height.

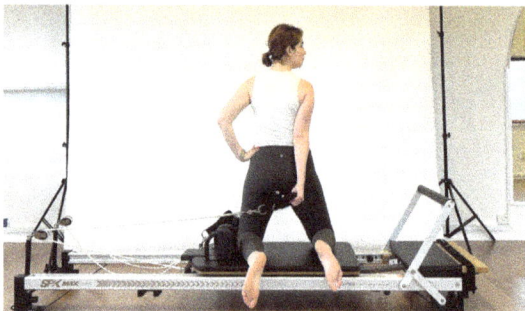

C
INHALE

1. Return to position **A**.
2. Repeat on the other side.

CORK BORER

Strength: Shoulder, arms, obliques

Level: Intermediate   **Repetition:** 8-10   **Springs:** Light to medium

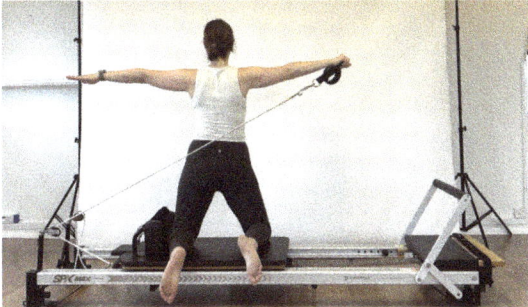

A
START

1. High kneeling facing sideways on the carriage with your legs shoulder width apart.
2. The footbar hand holds the back strap and both arms are placed at shoulder level out toward the sides.

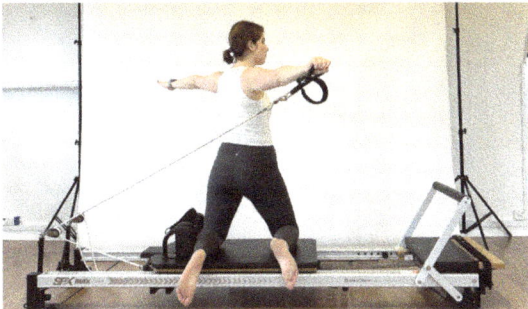

B
EXHALE

1. Twist your ribs. Your chest faces toward the footbar.

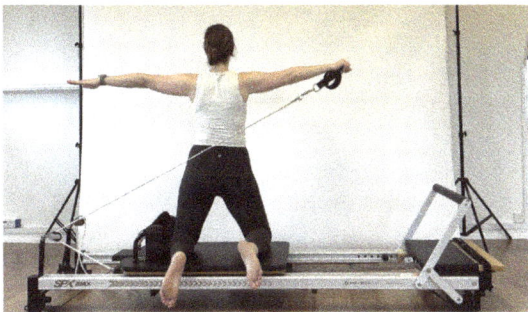

C
INHALE

1. Return to position **A**.
2. Repeat on the other side.

VARIATION

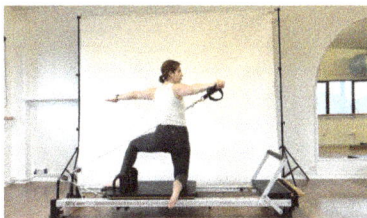

1. Place the shoulder rest foot on top of the headrest **(B)**

THE SCREWDRIVER PREP

Strength: Shoulder, arms, obliques

Level: Intermediate   **Repetition:** 8-10   **Springs:** Light to medium

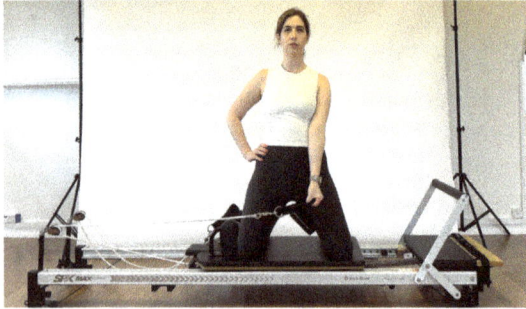

A
START

1. High kneeling facing sideways on the carriage with your legs shoulder width apart.
2. The footbar hand holds the front strap.

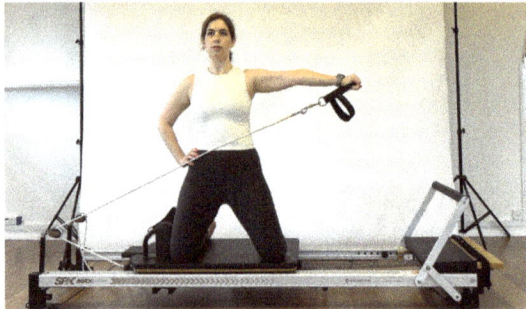

B
EXHALE

1. Lift your hand opening the arm sideways to shoulder level.

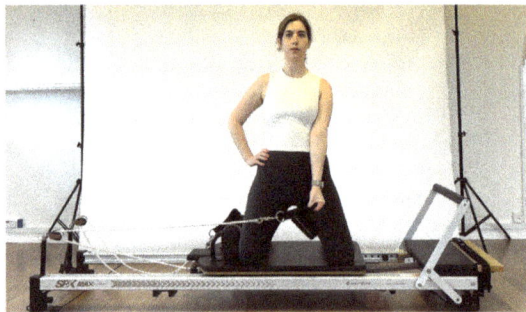

C
INHALE

1. Return to position **A**.
2. Repeat on the other side.

THE SCREWDRIVER

Strength: Shoulder, arms, obliques

Level: Intermediate **Repetition:** 8-10 **Springs:** Light to medium

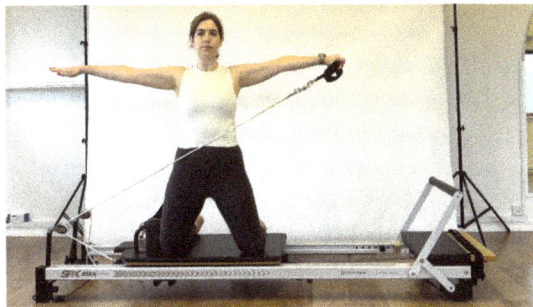

A
START

1. High kneeling facing sideways on the carriage with your legs shoulder width apart.
2. The footbar hand holds the front strap and both arms are placed at shoulder level out toward the sides.

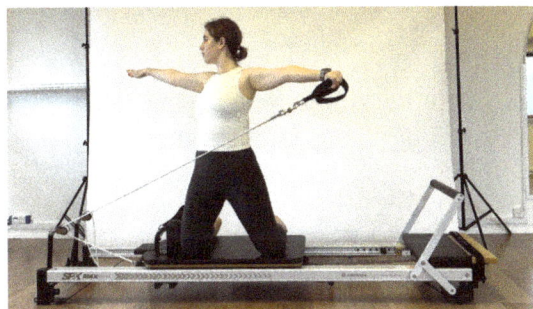

B
EXHALE

1. Twist your chest toward the risers.

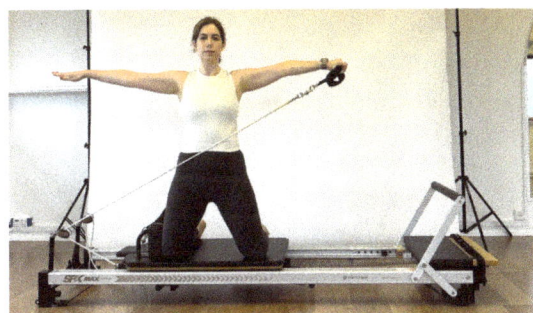

C
INHALE

1. Return to position **A**.
2. Repeat on the other side.

VARIATION

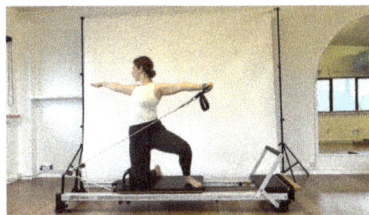

1. Place the foot closest to the footbar toward the front corner of the carriage **(B)**

HEART PIERCER I

Strength: Chest, shoulders, arms, obliques

Level: Intermediate   **Repetition:** 8-10   **Springs:** Light to medium

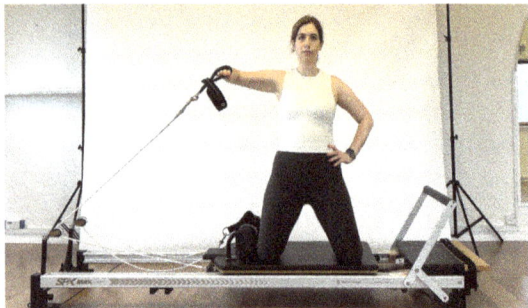

A
START

1. High kneeling facing sideways on the carriage with your legs shoulder width apart.
2. The riser hand holds the front strap with the elbow bent at 45 degrees.
3. The other hand is on the hip.

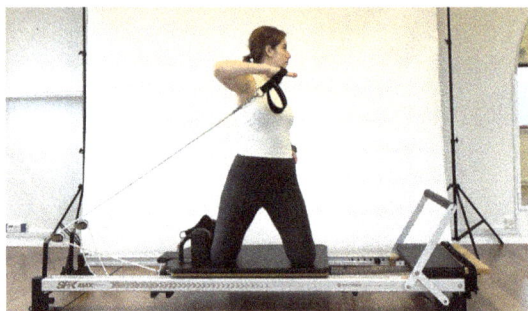

B
EXHALE

1. Pull your hand to your chest as you rotate your ribs to face the footbar.

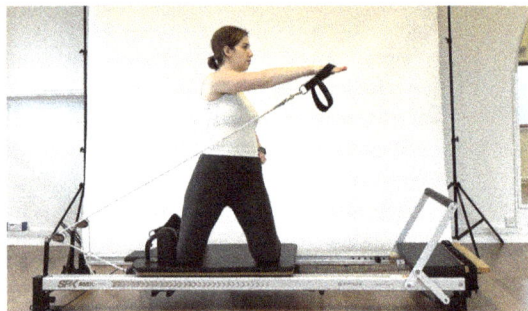

C
INHALE

1. Extend your arm toward the footbar.

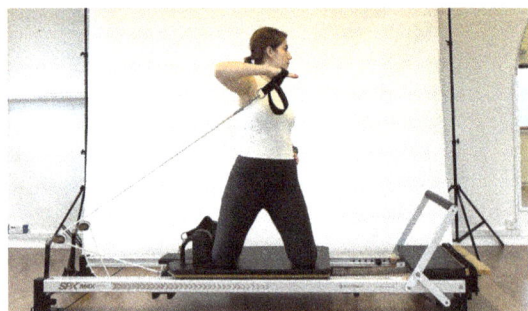

D
EXHALE

1. Return to position **B**.

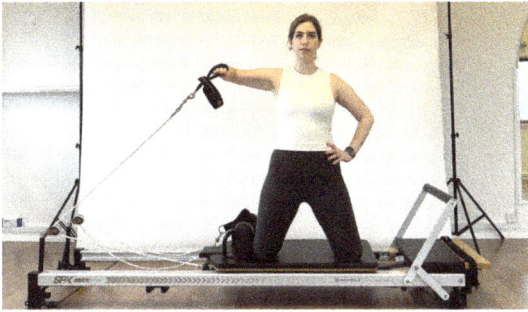

E
INHALE

1. Return to position **A**.
2. Repeat on the other side.

VARIATION 1

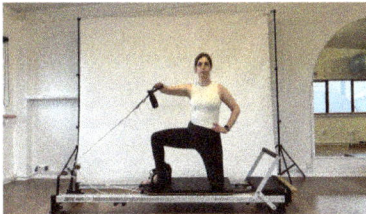

1. Place the riser leg toward the outside of the shoulder rest in external rotation with the foot on the carriage and knee bent. **(A)**

PROGRESSION

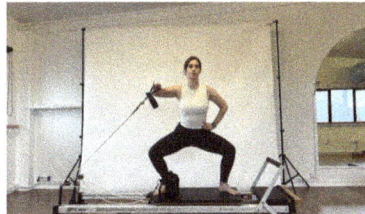

1. Stand on the carriage with both legs externally rotated and placed as wide as the carriage will allow. The knees are bent. **(A)**

HEART PIERCER II

Strength: Chest, shoulders, arms,obliques

Level: Intermediate   **Repetition:** 8-10   **Springs:** Medium

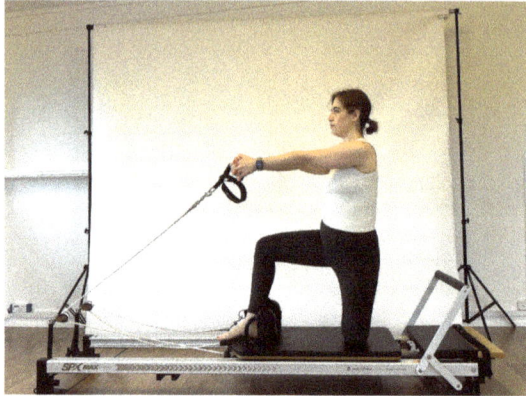

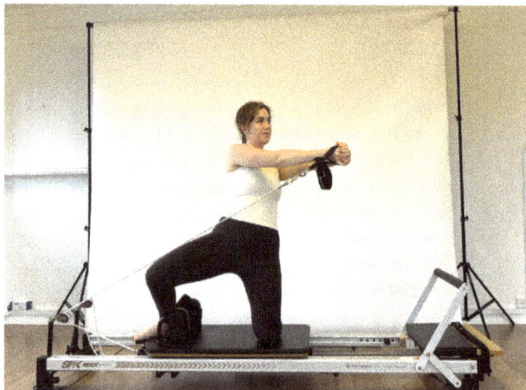

A
START

1. Kneel sideways on the carriage with one leg in external rotation and the foot on the outer edge of the carriage next to the shoulder rest.
2. The other knee is under the hip and aligned with shoulder rest. The foot is at the edge of the carriage.
3. Both hands hold one strap. Keep the elbows straight and rotate toward the turned out leg.

B
EXHALE

1. Rotate your ribs to the other side.

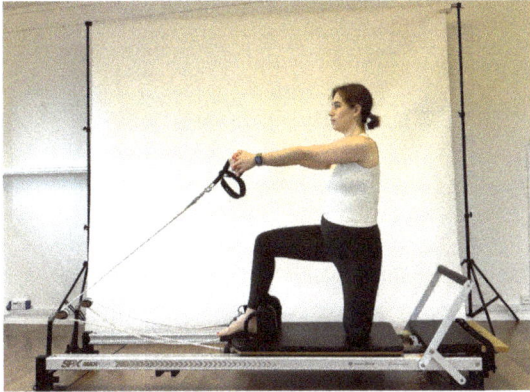

C
INHALE

1. Return to position **A**.
2. Repeat on the other side.

PROGRESSION

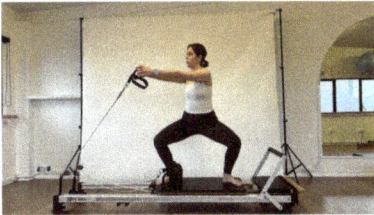

1. Stand on top of the carriage with both
   legs in external rotation and knees bent. **(A)**

TIPPY TOE I

Strength: Chest, back, shoulders, obliques, quads, inner thighs

Level: Intermediate   **Repetition:** 8-10   **Springs:** Medium

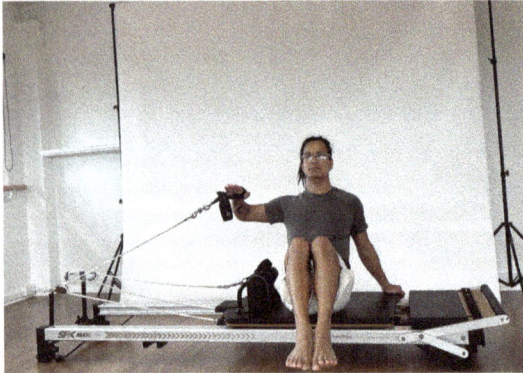

A
START

1. Sitting at the edge of the carriage with your spine in flexion. Both legs are lifted off the floor and pressed together.
2. The hand closest to the footbar rests on the back corner of the carriage. The other hand holds the strap with the palm facing the floor and the elbow bent at 90 degrees to the side of your body.

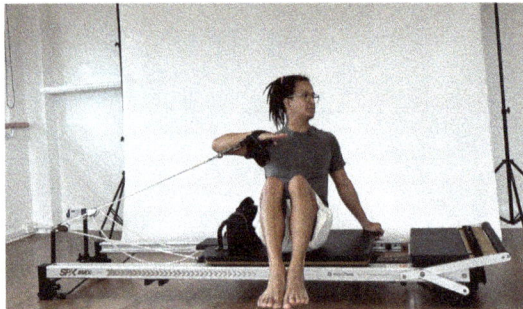

B
EXHALE

1. Pull the strap bringing the arm in front of your chest and start rotating your ribs.
2. Look toward the side you are twisting to.

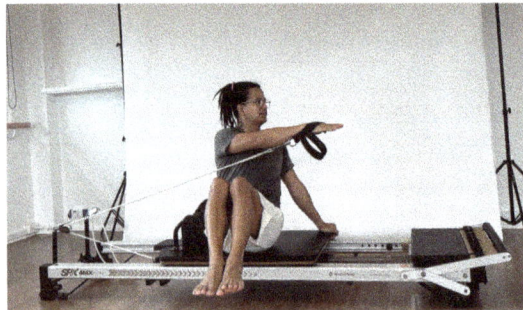

C
INHALE

1. Continue twisting and extend your elbow. Your fingers point toward the footbar.

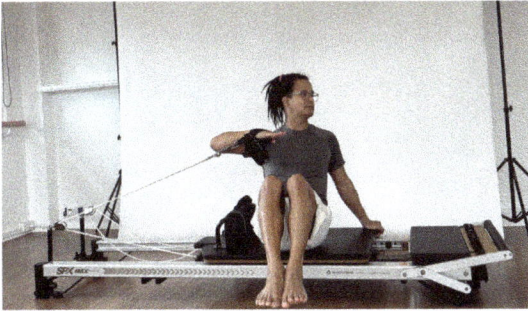

D
EXHALE

1. Return to position **B**.

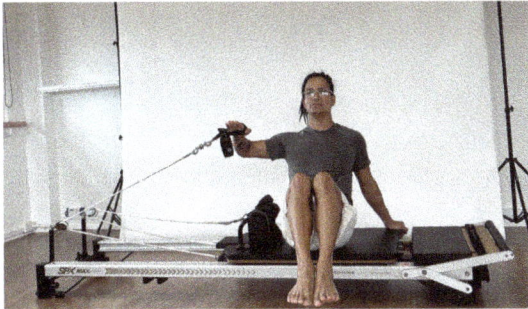

E
INHALE

1. Return to position **A**.
2. Repeat on the other side.

PROGRESSION

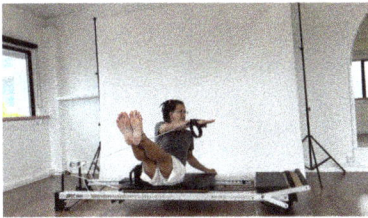

1. Extend both legs into a Teaser position **(C)**

TIPPY TOE II

Strength: chest, shoulder, oblique, quads, inner thigh

Level: Intermediate   **Repetition:** 8-10   **Springs:** Medium

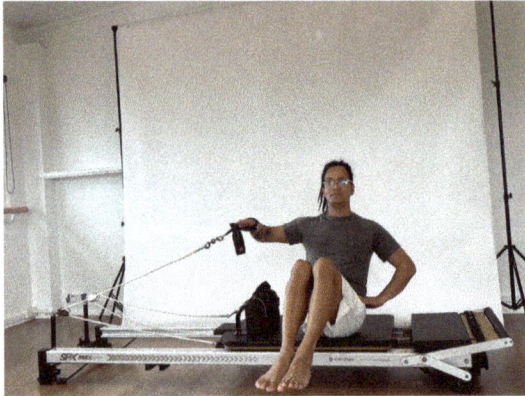

A
START

1. Sitting at the edge of the carriage with your spine in flexion. Both legs are lifted off the floor and pressed together.
2. The hand closest to the footbar rests on your hip. The other hand holds the strap with the palm facing the floor and the elbow bent at 90 degrees to the side of your body.

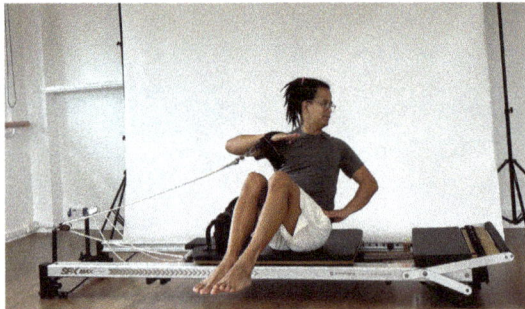

B
EXHALE

1. Pull the strap bringing the arm in front of your chest and start rotating your ribs.
2. Look toward the side you are twisting to.

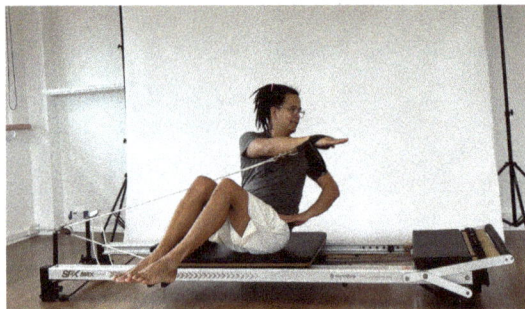

C
INHALE

1. Continue twisting and extend your elbow. Your fingers point toward the footbar.

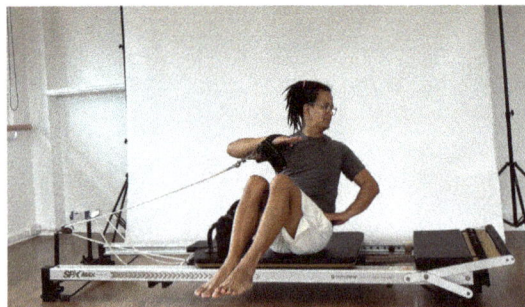

D
EXHALE

1. Return to position **B**.

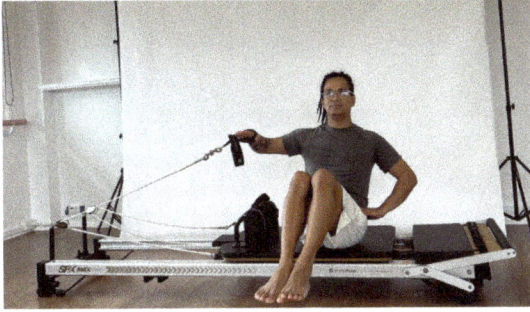

E
INHALE

1. Return to position **A**
2. Repeat on the other side

PROGRESSION

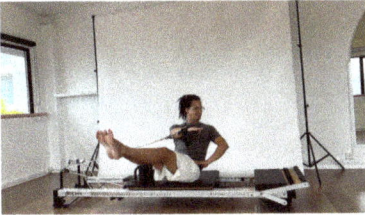

1. Extend both legs out to a Teaser position **(C)**

TIPPY TOE III

Strength: Chest, shoulders, obliques, quads, inner thighs

Level: Intermediate   **Repetition:** 8-10   **Springs:** Medium

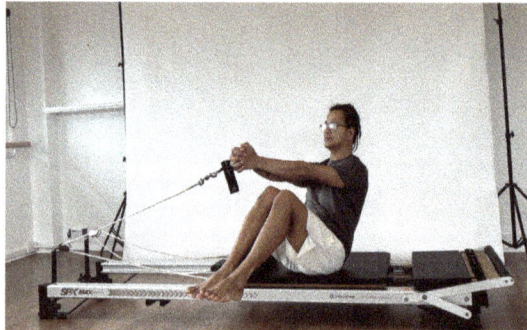

A
START

1. Sitting at the edge of the carriage with your spine in flexion. Both legs are lifted off the floor and pressed together.
2. Hold onto the strap with both hands clasped together. Extend your arms in front of you at shoulder height. Twist your ribs toward the risers.

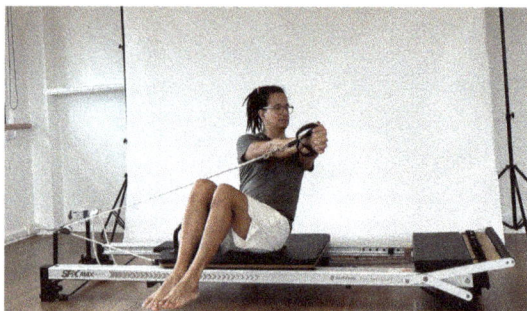

B
EXHALE

1. Rotate towards the footbar pulling the strap and rotating your ribs in the same direction.

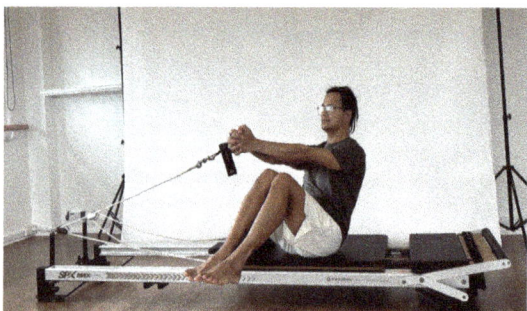

C
INHALE

1. Return to position **A**.
2. Repeat on the other side

BASEMENT I

Strength: Chest, shoulders, arms, obliques, inner thighs

Level: Intermediate   **Repetition:** 8-10   **Springs:** Medium

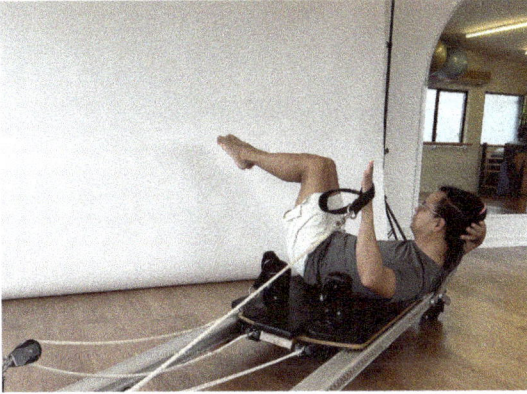

A
START

1. Lie on your back on the carriage with one side lining up next to the shoulder rests.
2. Place your legs in table top and lift your head and chest into an abdominal curl position.
3. Hold onto one strap with the shoulder rest side hand. Bend the elbow and point your fingers up to the ceiling.
4. Support your head with the other hand.

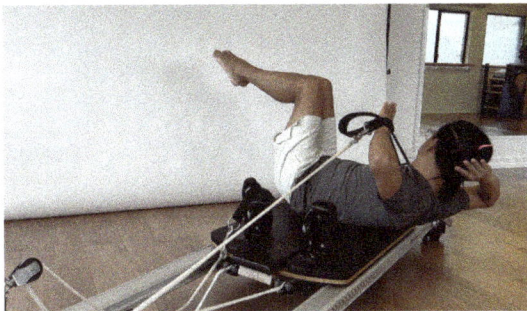

B
EXHALE

1. Twist your spine toward the footbar slightly as you pull your arm toward your chest.

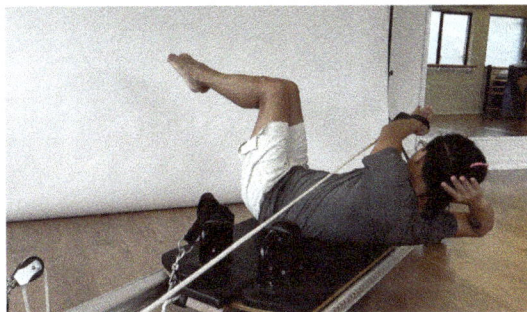

C
INHALE

1. Extend your elbow, reaching your hand to the footbar.

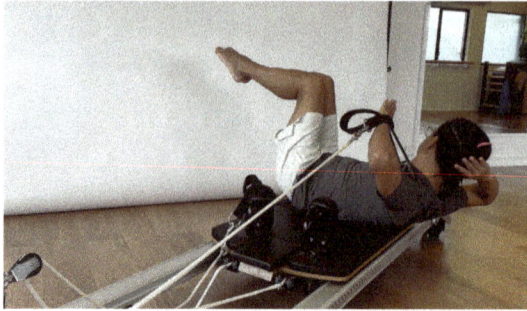

D

EXHALE

1. Return to position **B**.

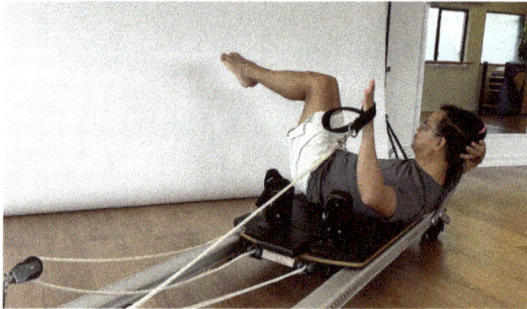

E

INHALE

1. Return to position **A**
2. Repeat on the other side.

PROGRESSION 1

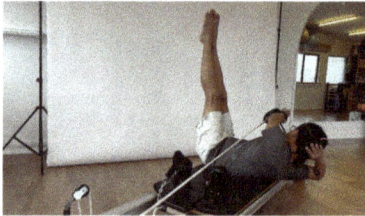

1. Extend both legs to 90 degrees **(C)**

PROGRESSION 2

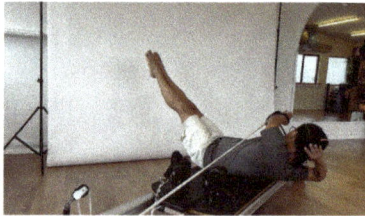

1. Extend both legs to 45 degrees **(C)**

PROGRESSION 3

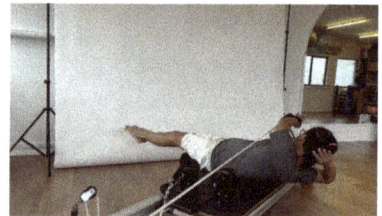

1. Extend both legs 180 degrees **(C)**

BASEMENT II

Strength: Chest, shoulders, arms, obliques, inner thighs

Level: Intermediate   **Repetition:** 8-10   **Springs:** Medium

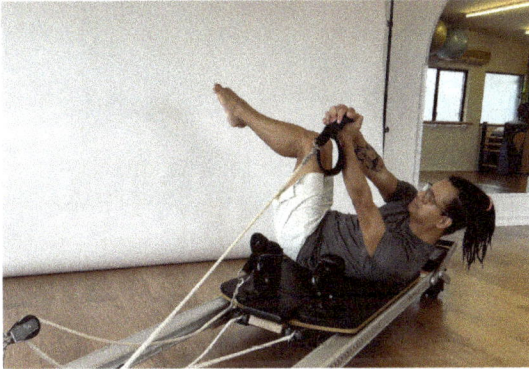

A
START

1. Lie on your back on the carriage with one side lining up next to the shoulder rests.
2. Place your legs in table top and lift your head and chest into an abdominal curl position.
3. Hold onto one strap with both hands. Extend your elbows and interlace your fingers around the strap.

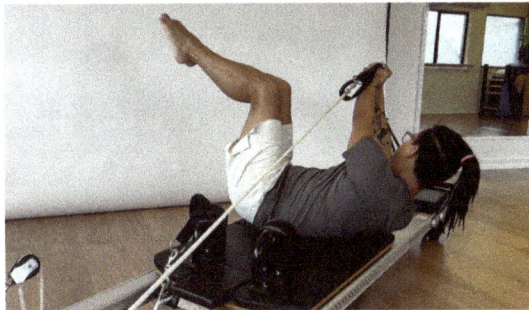

B
EXHALE

1. Twist your chest and head towards the footbar as you pull the strap across your chest below shoulder level.

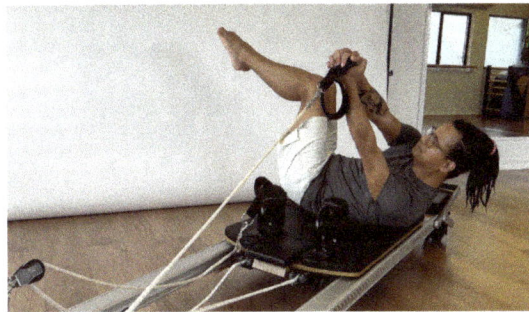

C
INHALE

1. Return to position **A**.
2. Repeat on the other side.

PROGRESSION 1

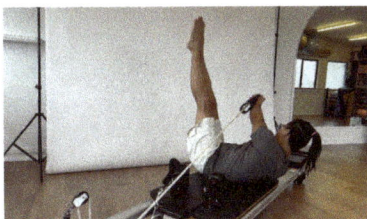

1. Extend both legs to 90 degrees **(C)**

PROGRESSION 2

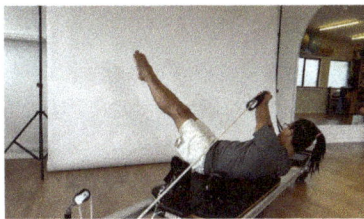

1. Extend both legs to 45 degrees **(C)**

PROGRESSION 3

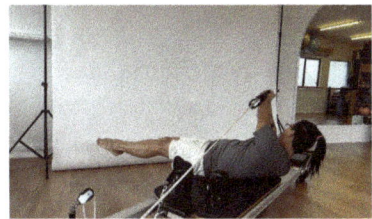

1. Extend both legs to 180 degrees **(C)**

OPEN STAGE

Strength: Chest ,shoulders,arms, tricep, abs

Level: Intermediate **Repetition:** 8-10 **Springs:** Light to medium

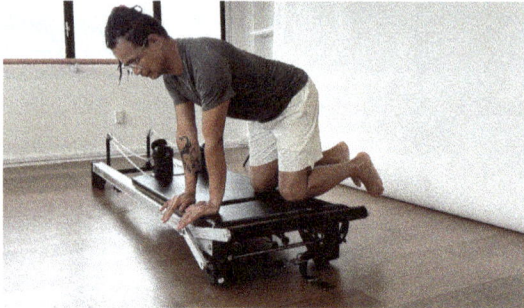

A
START

1. Four point kneeling position sideways across the carriage.
2. Place one hand and foot on the standing platform and the other hand and foot on the corner of the carriage.

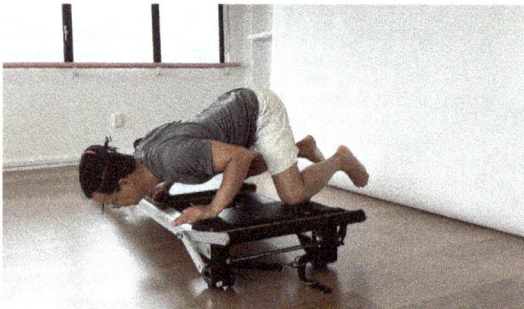

B
EXHALE

1. Open the carriage as wide as your shoulders.
2. Bend your elbows bringing your chest closer to the frame.

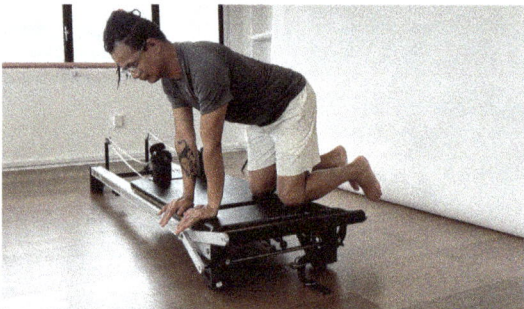

C
INHALE

1. Return to position **A**.
2. Repeat on the other side.

PROGRESSION 1

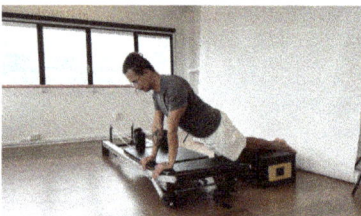

1. Kneeling plank position with your knees on the reformer box and the knees on top of the box **(A)**

PROGRESSION 2

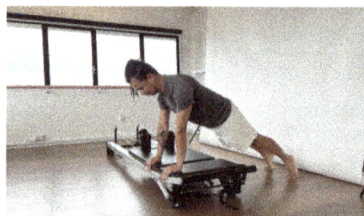

1. Plank position with your legs extended out behind you on the floor **(A)**

CYCLONE PREP

Strength: Shoulder, obliques, glutes, quads,hamstrings, inner thighs

Level: Intermediate   **Repetition:** 8-10   **Springs:** Medium

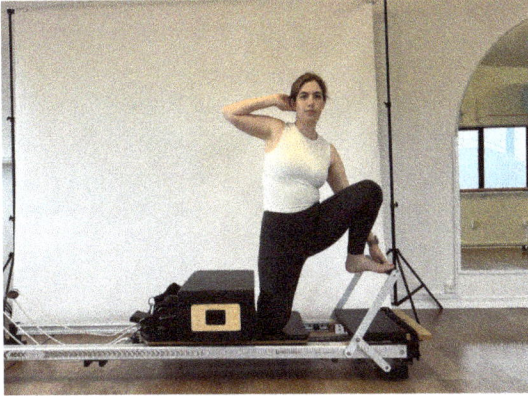

A
START

1. Place the reformer box across the front of the shoulder rests.
2. Kneel on the carriage with one knee next to the box and the other foot elevated on the reformer footbar at the corner of the bar and externally rotated.
3. Place the riser hand behind your head and side flex your spine toward the footbar.
4. The other hand holds the middle of the footbar.

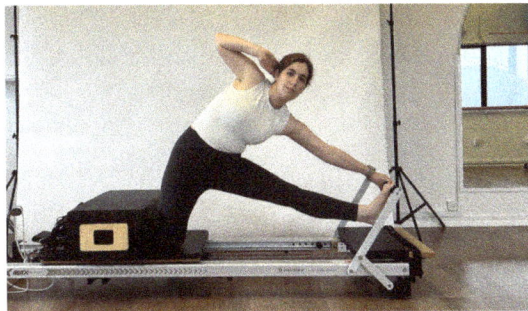

B
EXHALE

1. Push the carriage out extending your footbar knee until you feel a stretch along the inner thigh.

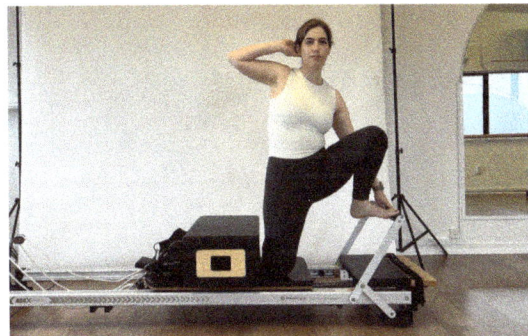

C
INHALE

1. Return to position **A**.
2. Repeat on the other side.

CYCLONE I

Strength: Shoulder, obliques, glutes, quads, inner thighs

Level: Intermediate   **Repetition:** 8-10   **Springs:** Medium

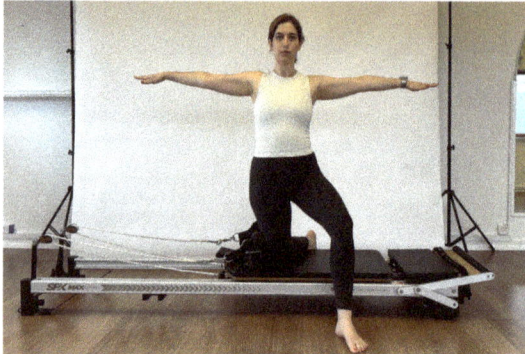

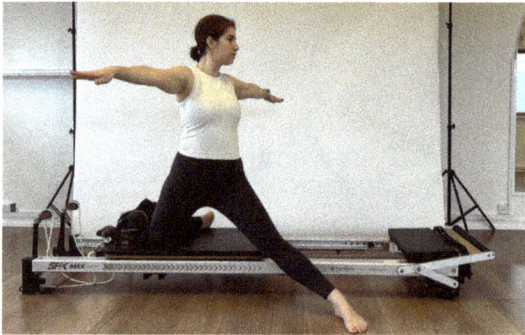

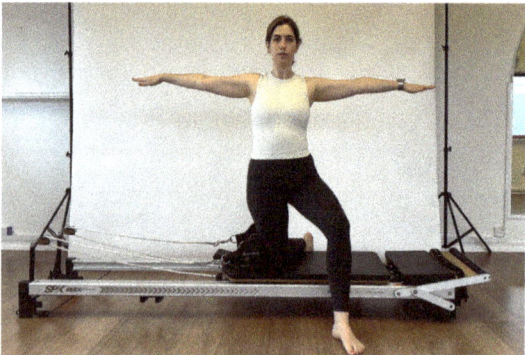

A
START

1. Stand in front of the side of the reformer. Kneel with one knee in front of the shoulder rests. The other foot is on the floor with a 45 degree turn out and the knee bent
2. Reach both arms out to the side in a T-shape.

B
EXHALE

1. Push your legs away from each other as your spine rotates toward the footbar. Extend the knee of your standing leg.

C
INHALE

1. Return to position **A**.
2. Repeat on the other side.

PROGRESSION 1

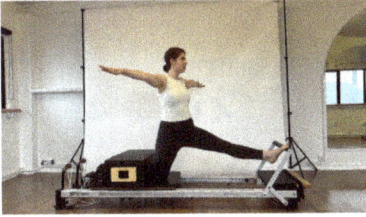

1. Kneel next to the reformer box in the short box position. The other foot on the footbar toward the front corner and externally rotated **(A)**

PROGRESSION 2

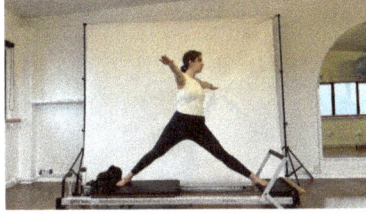

1. Stand on the carriage with one foot on the standing platform and the other wedged against the shoulder rest **(B)**

PROGRESSION 3

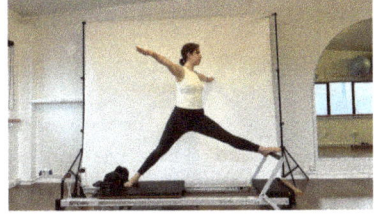

1. Stand on the carriage with one foot on the footbar and the other wedged against the shoulder rest **(B)**

CYCLONE II

Strength: Shoulder, obliques, glutes, quads, inner thigh

Level: Intermediate   **Repetition:** 8-10   **Springs:** Medium

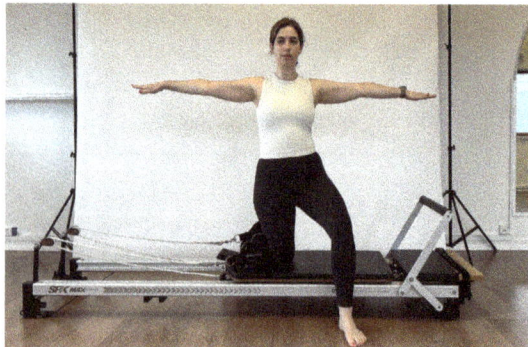

A
START

1. Stand in front of the side of the reformer. Kneel with one knee in front of the shoulder rests. The other foot is on the floor with a 45 degree turn out and the knee bent
2. Reach both arms out to the side in a T-shape.

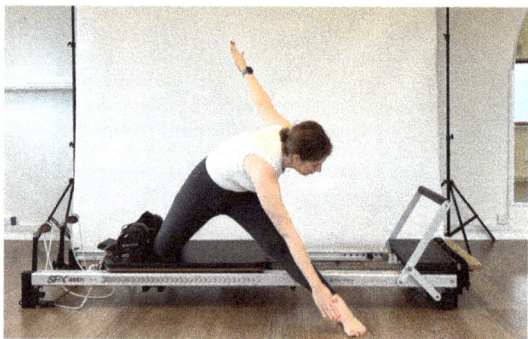

B
EXHALE

1. As your legs separate, twist and reach down toward the floor leg's foot.
2. Bring your hand to the outside of the foot.

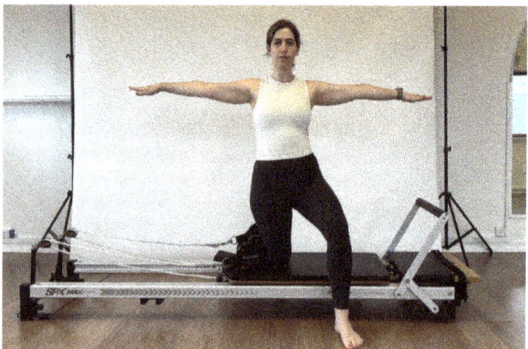

C
INHALE

1. Return to position **A**.
2. Repeat on the other side.

PROGRESSION 1

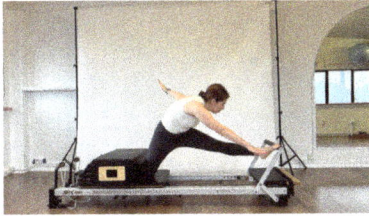

1. Kneel next to the reformer box in the short box position. The other foot on the footbar toward the front corner and externally rotated **(A)**

PROGRESSION 2

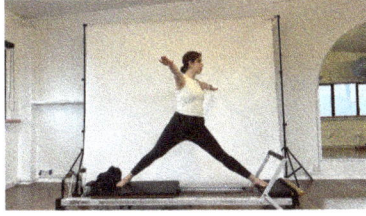

1. Stand on the carriage with one foot on the standing platform and the other wedged against the shoulder rest **(B)**

PROGRESSION 3

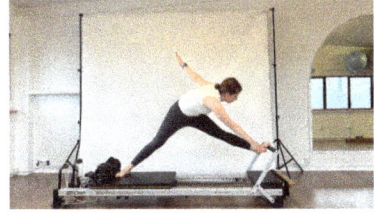

1. Stand on the carriage with one foot on the footbar and the other wedged against the shoulder rest **(B)**

QUEEN'S LANDING I

Strength: Glutes, quads

Level: Beginners   **Repetition:** 8-10   **Springs:** Medium

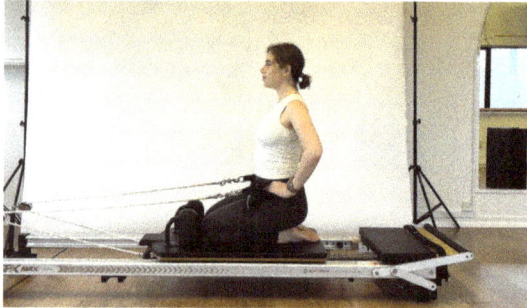

A
START

1. Japanese style kneel on the carriage facing the risers.
2. Your knees touch the shoulder rests.
3. Hold onto the straps and place your hands on your hips.

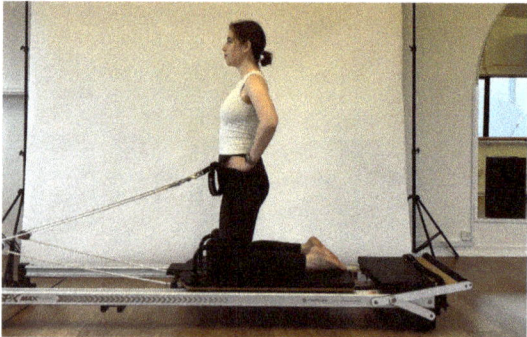

B
EXHALE

1. Lift your hips into a high kneel.
2. Keep your spine as vertical as possible.

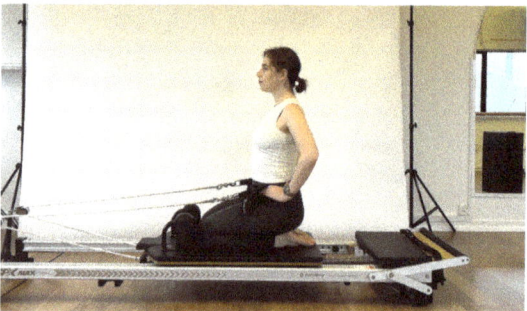

C
INHALE

1. Return to position **A**.

VARIATION

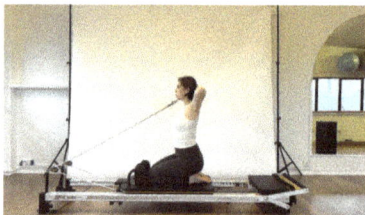

1. Place your hands behind your head, and the strap around your elbows **(A)**

QUEEN'S LANDING II

Strength: Glutes, quads

Level: Intermediate   **Repetition:** 8-10   **Springs:** Medium

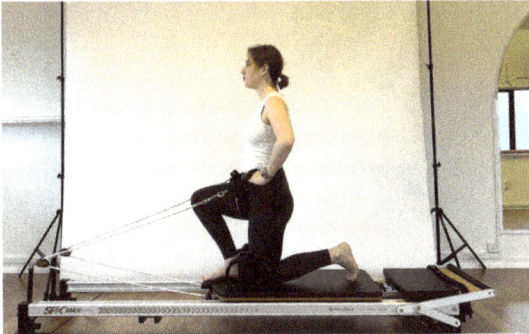

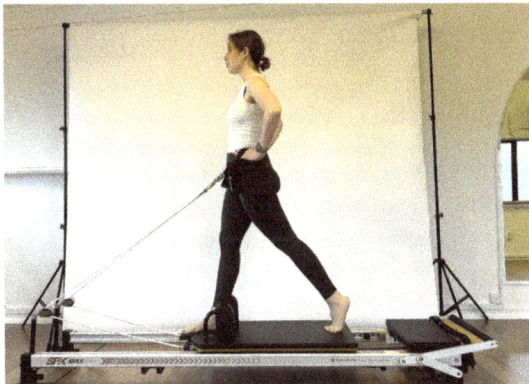

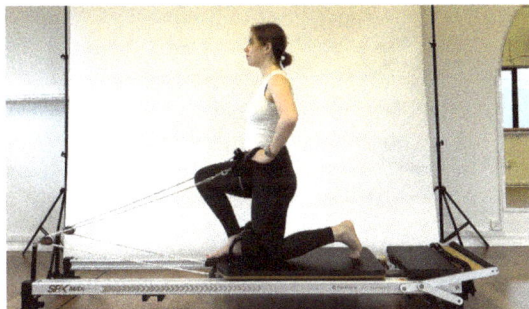

A
START

1. Kneel on the carriage with one knee against the shoulder rest and the other on the headrest
2. Tuck your toes under of the kneeling leg to give more stability
3. Hold onto the straps and place your hands onto your hips.

B
EXHALE

1. Stand up with control using your back leg to push off with.
2. Keep your spine as vertical as possible.

C
INHALE

1. Return to position **A**.
2. Repeat on the other side.

BROOKE'S LUNGE I

Strength: Quads, hip flexors

Level: Intermediate   **Repetition:** 8-10   **Springs:** Light to medium

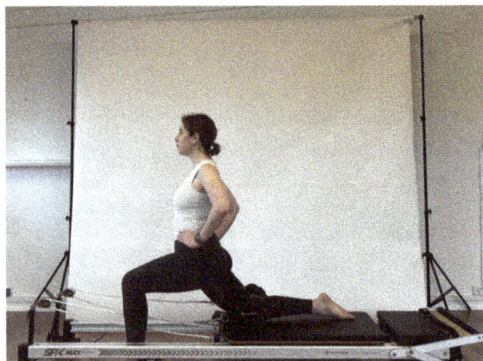

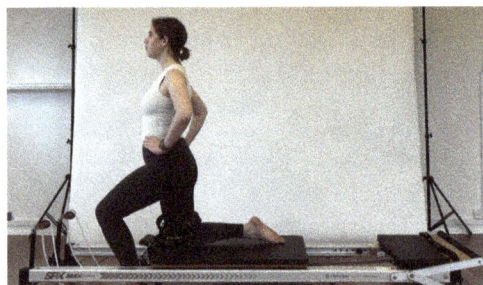

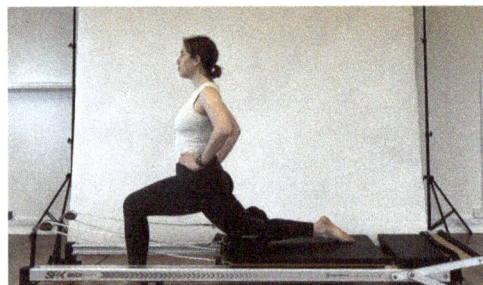

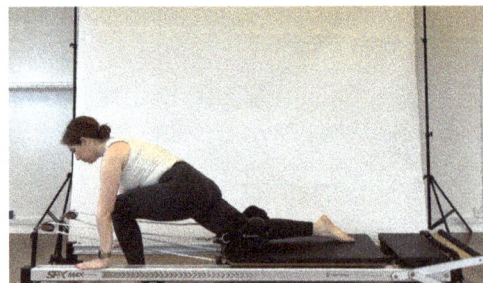

A
START

1. Stand next to the carriage facing the risers. Your spine is in neutral alignment.
2. Place the leg closest to the reformer on the carriage with the toes tucked under. Bring your hip into extension, opening the front of the hip into a lunge.
3. The other foot stands on the floor. Bend the knee to 90 degrees and press the leg against the frame.

B
EXHALE

1. Pull your back knee toward the front leg until your carriage knee is under your hip. The floor knee straightens to allow you to do the movement.

C
INHALE

1. Return to position **A**.
2. Repeat on the other side.

MODIFICATION

1. Place your hands on the frame.

BROOKE'S LUNGE II

Strength: Quads, hip flexors

Level: Intermediate   **Repetition:** 8-10   **Springs:** Light to medium

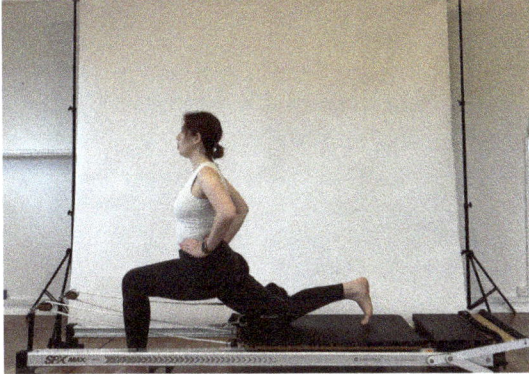

A
START

1. Stand next to the carriage facing the risers. Your spine is in neutral alignment.
2. Place the leg closest to the reformer on the carriage with the toes tucked under. Bring your hip into extension, opening the front of the hip into a lunge.
3. The other foot stands on the floor. Bend the knee to 90 degrees and press the leg against the frame.

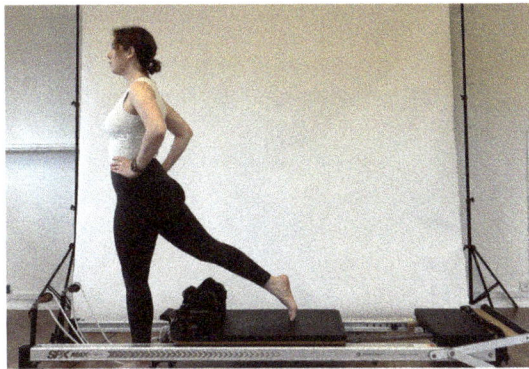

B
EXHALE

1. Straighten your floor knee while pulling your back leg towards the front leg.

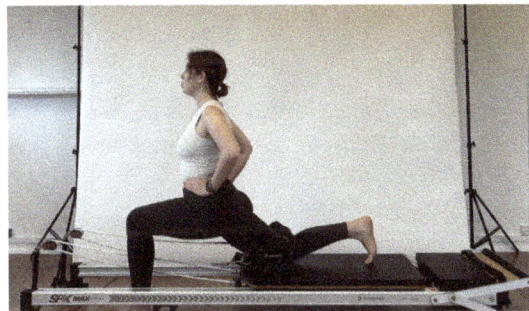

C
INHALE

1. Return to position **A**.
2. Repeat on the other side.

KNEELING KNIGHT I

Strength: Inner thighs, hamstrings, calves

Level: Intermediate   **Repetition:** 8-10   **Springs:** Light to medium

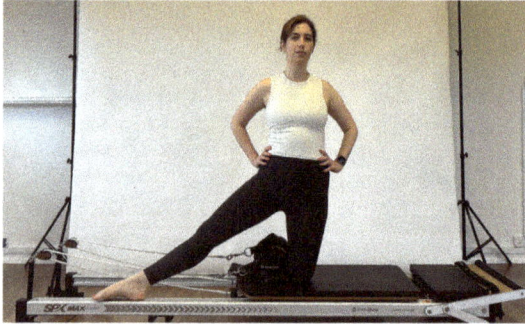

A
START

1. Kneel sideways on the carriage. Place one leg along the inside of the shoulder rests. The other leg is extended and the foot is resting on the frame.
2. Place your hands on your hips

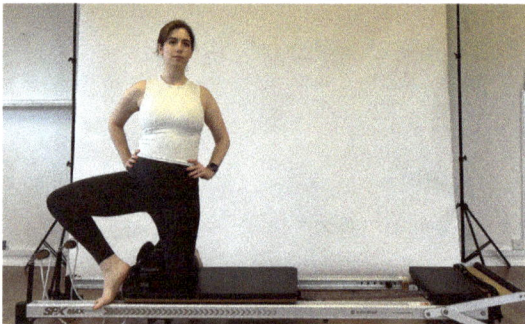

B
EXHALE

1. Pull the carriage toward the frame leg. Bend the knee and lift the frame leg's heel off the frame as you bring the carrier closer.

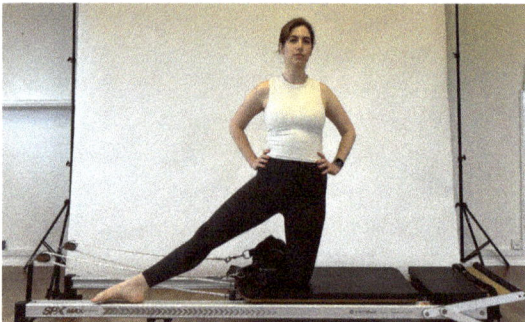

C
INHALE

1. Return to position **A**.
2. Repeat on the other side.

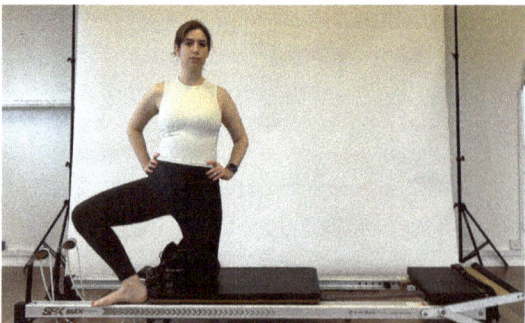

MODIFICATION
1. Keep your heel down.

KNEELING KNIGHT II

Strength: Inner thighs, hamstrings, calves

Level: Intermediate   **Repetition:** 8-10   **Springs:** Light to medium

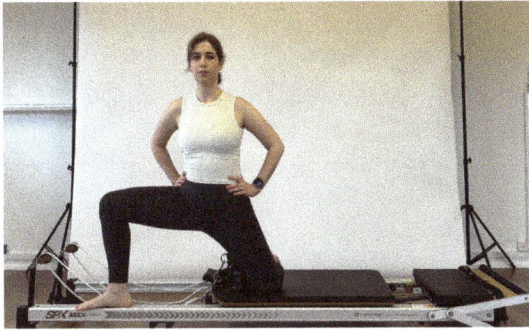

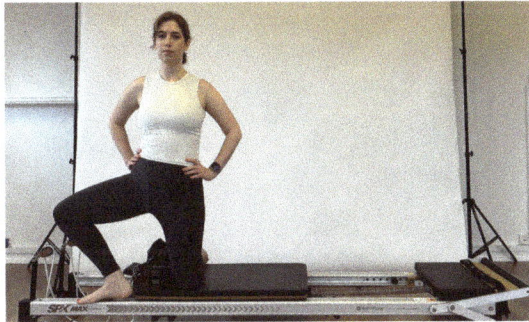

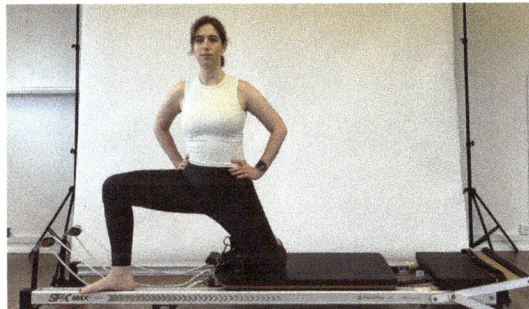

A
START

1. Kneel on the carriage. Place one leg against the inside of the shoulder rests. The other leg is on the frame in an external rotation.
2. Lunge your body weight over toward the frame leg.
3. Place your hands on your hips.

B
EXHALE

1. Pull the carriage toward your frame leg until your knee is under your hip.

C
INHALE

1. Return to position **A**.
2. Repeat on the other side.

PROGRESSION

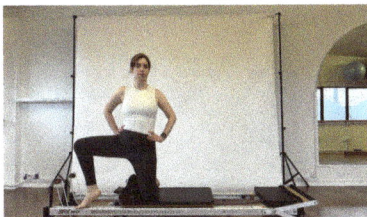

1. Lift the frame leg's heel off and balance on the ball of your foot **(B)**

KNEELING KNIGHT III

Strength: Inner thighs, quad, glutess

Level: Intermediate   **Repetition:** 8-10   **Springs:** Light to medium

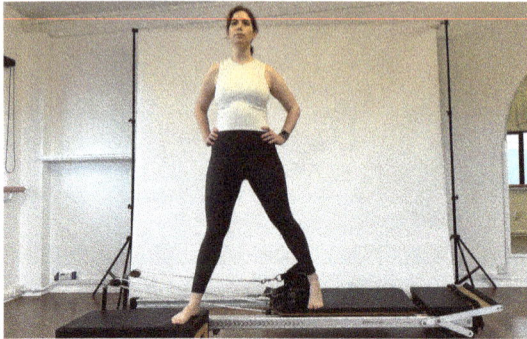

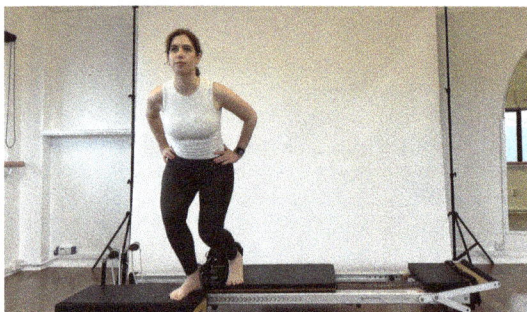

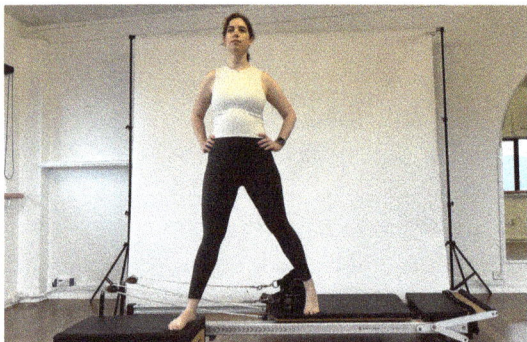

A
START

1. Place the reformer box next to the riser end of the reformer on the floor. Stand on the box with one foot. Place the other foot on the inside of the shoulder rest.
2. Both legs are straight.
3. Place your hands on your hips.

B
EXHALE

1. As you pull the carriage in with the shoulder rest leg, hinge at your hips like a half squat.

C
INHALE

1. Return to position **A**.
2. Repeat on the other side.

PROGRESSION

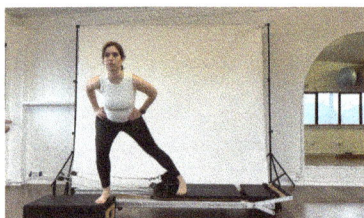

1. Maintain the squat position **(A)**

www.ingramcontent.com/pod-product-compliance
Lightning Source LLC
Chambersburg PA
CBHW051313020426
42333CB00028B/3317